Natural to Supernatural Health

David Herzog

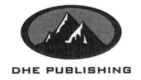

DHE PUBLISHING

Dedication

This book is dedicated to the Creator of Heaven and Earth for leading me in the direction of Natural to Super Natural Health and giving me the courage, motivation, and inspiration to write and finish this book. I will spend the rest of my life exploring the depths of the Creator and His wonderful Creation and share it to the world.

Contents

Introduction

TRANSFORM YOUR BODY INTO A LEAN, MEAN, SUPER-ENERGIZED BEING

Everybody wants to look and feel their best! I know because I have talked with, counseled, and helped people around the world from every sphere of life including single moms, heads of state, actors and entertainers, athletes, construction workers, business leaders, spiritual seekers, students, and people on every continent and sphere of society. People want the same thing: a thin, vibrant, energetic, youthful, radiating, clear-skinned, super-healthy, bliss-ful, toned, and muscular body. They want to be so super-charged and live stress-free not only with health and a fabulous body, but they want to know sheer joy and peace inside and out while liv-ing out their destiny and dreams instead of just existing. Imagine having all that and being connected to the Highest Power Source of love and peace, all at the same time!

Does that sound like what you are looking for? Does it some-times feel there are physical, mental, emotional, and spiritual blockages that keep you in a stagnant stage of going through the motions, as if there were invisible barriers somehow stopping you from having the willpower to go from existing to thriving in every area of life? Does this constant cycle keep you feeling sluggish and at times frustrated that your body is not getting any younger or thinner no matter what you try, affecting your actions of pursuing your life-long dreams? Have you ever thought that if you could just lose those extra pounds and be super-healthy you could have the courage to also tackle achieving your greatest desires? Well it is not only possible but easier to realize than ever before due to the advanced knowledge you are about to read in this book.

This book will take you from a natural to a super natural and super-energized state that will totally create a more attractive and charismatic countenance, a healthier and leaner body, drastic change in appearance and youthfulness, an entirely new mental outlook on life, and a stress-free and carefree standard of living like you always wanted deep down inside.

FROM NATURAL TO SUPER NATURAL

When you start to drop the excess pounds and cleanse your body, eat living raw and organic foods, super-energize your body, look 10 to 20 years younger, and change your outlook on life, something else begins to happen. On a physical level, things are very different but then you start to tap into another spiritual plane. All of a sudden, you are just going for a nature walk when suddenly a sense of sheer love, joy, energy, peace, and happiness start to flood your entire being. Not only are the high energy raw, natural, and organic foods releasing high levels of nutrients and energy, but because your newly cleansed and energized body has been unclogged and is now fully alive, you also start to be more aware of the invisible world around you. You start to simply feel sheer bliss just to be alive, being thankful for the beauty all around you. Once you have removed years of undesired toxins and waste in your body, you become a channel to receive immense levels of energy, joy, and peace. Thankfulness for life itself starts to overtake you effortlessly.

The principles in this book will start to work for you immediately so you don't have to wait until you are finished with the book, but you can start to apply the keys and lifestyle changes right away from chapter to chapter. Go ahead and get excited about your new life that is just around the corner!

FROM DEATH TO LIFE!

Once you delve into this book and experience the sheer ecstasy of your new life, you will never want to go back! You will feel as if you came back from the dead when you think back to how you used to feel and live.

So many people are confused by the myriad of claims from so many supplements, commercials, and products that claim to be the solution for energy, skin beauty, and health that leads to more frustration once you realize these were empty promises.

Once you get a hold of the truth and understand health at its core and live out your new lifestyle change, you will never again be easily swayed by the latest fad nor will you run to the nearest pharmacy to be experimented on by the latest drugs with major side effects. You will have the confidence and evidence of a truly super natural and super-energized body vibrating on much higher frequencies than most people. The moment you walk into a room, people will notice something powerful emanating from the inside out of you. Besides the glowing skin and radiating healthy body, people will notice a truly transformed human being enjoying the highest possible state of health in mind, body, and spirit.

HOW THIS BOOK WILL CHANGE YOUR LIFE

There are many health books out there on the market. Some focus on raw organic foods, others focus on cleansing, while others focus on exercise. Some even tell you about the latest scientific breakthroughs in health, medicine, and anti-aging. Still others will focus more on the spiritual side of the human experience and how this affects your health.

After having researched, studied, and lived for health in every possible way most of my adult life, I have endeavored to give it all to you in one book in an easy-to-read and motivational matter so you can get started right away. I have come to the conclusion that the only way to truly achieve *Super Natural Health* is to take a multi-pronged approach and hit it all at once on all levels while exploring the latest cutting edge discoveries in natural, raw, and organic health that are simply mind-boggling and life-changing.

Whether you are simply needing a weight loss cure that really works, more stamina and energy, wanting to change your diet with miracle raw organic superfoods and exercise, tap into the latest natural anti-aging secrets and ways to rebalance your hormones naturally at any age, find the solution to your teeth problems, or reprogram your life for total success and be connected to the highest power source, you are on the right track as you are reading this book not by chance but guided by divine destiny as you will discover truths you never knew about before. Get ready for the change of a lifetime!

Chapter 1

Cleansing

"What you get by achieving your goals is not as important as what you become by achieving your goals."
—Zig Ziglar

To begin your journey from natural to super natural health, the first step is cleansing. As your body begins to cleanse itself of toxins—impurities and "stuff"—it will suddenly begin to function at optimal super charged levels. You will see yourself go from natural to super natural health as you tap into infinite possibilities—not just physically but mentally, emotionally, and spiritually.

You have heard the expression: *What goes up must come down.* Well it is equally true that: *What goes in must come out.* The problem is that much of what most people eat today does not all come out of our bodies but stays and rots inside our intestines, which starts complications.

When you eat food that is alive and vibrant, organic, and raw, you start to feel the same energy level of that food. When you consume fresh organic, raw food; you internally feel cleaner, lighter, less burdened. This affects your emotions, energy level, and desire for the supernatural. When you eat "dead foods" robbed of nutrition and life, that death process starts to affect your body and your life including your mind, will, emotions, and everything else.

When you are in a natural setting—the mountains or the ocean—you not only feel more inclined to eat better and exercise you also become more spiritual and more prone to pray, meditate, sing, and explore the spiritual world. This is because the blockages of tiredness, stress, and manmade surroundings have been removed. In the same way, when your body takes in raw nutrients in their most natural form, these nutrients release a much higher energy, leave you feeling euphoric, and help you heal. When you eat manmade food that has been processed, the atoms and soundwaves of food particles are broken down—not to mention the nutritional qualities—leaving you less energized.

When you are often tired, sluggish, easily annoyed, or stressed, these are indicators that you are most likely blocked and clogged in several ways and not getting that direct energy high that you could. Healthy eating and living can be one pathway to release yourself into higher realms of health and the supernatural. Through healthy eating and living, you can go from natural to super natural health!

DETOX AND CLEANSING

As the seasons change, many people get the flu and colds. This is your body telling you it is time to detox and flush out the impurities. If you do this willingly, you don't have to experience the same "forced detox" that nature seems to bring upon us when we are overloaded. I often do a fast or cleanse at the start of a new season and I notice that I don't get affected by whatever new virus or flu that comes around.

Healing can occur during cleansing and detox. Often, as one starts to do this cleansing process in the body, other areas—emotional, mental, and spiritual—will also experience a detox. All that is negative will start to flush out or come to the surface.

Most people in the western world have parasites, candida—intestines that are bloated because of undigested meats still in the gut and stomach lining that are putrefying the entire system and the list goes on. The entire body needs a full cleanse to begin the journey of super natural health. This includes the liver, gall bladder, colon, and skin. As you detox, you will start to notice a radical transformation: You will be filled with youthful vigor and energy and you will appear younger. Your skin and complexion will glow, you will experience weight loss, thickened hair, and an overall light feeling that you have not felt since childhood. Everyone will notice your positive outlook.

Once all your toxins and blockers are cleansed out of your system, you will start to radiate like never before as nothing will be slowing or stopping you blocking the energy paths.

You will start to tap into super energy and even supernatural realms that were not accessible when you were weighed down by the obstructions. Your mind will be much clearer as everything is now unclogged. Your emotions will also be much more balanced. A clean body radiates life, light, and joy and is very attractive to other people. Others are drawn to you when you are in this new state of cleansing and health.

Your body will go from survival and decay to actually being able to rebuild itself now that it is clean. Your body's energy will be able to work on healing and rebuilding instead of being over-burdened with toxins. Certain ailments and sicknesses often just vanish—certain allergies and the like.

One of the best and most thorough ways that I know of today to start the major cleansing process is to start with colon hydrotherapy.

Colon Hydrotherapy

This accelerates the detox process and will add years to your life. This helps to quickly detox without hindering your daily life as opposed to a slow detox and having to deal with extreme symptoms. It is simple, painless, and discreet. Just find a licensed colon therapist, as colonics are vital to your health in the day and age we live in to thoroughly eliminate impacted fecal matter and toxins. The ancients used this process for thousands of years. A series (anywhere from 6 to 12) of colonics at least once or twice a year is a good start.

The goal is to empty out your bladder, colon, liver, and intestines from years of backed up fecal matter and decay rotting in your body from undigested food—usually meats. This will allow your lymph system to drain. The other important thing is that you will be flushing out encrusted mucus, which poisons your system and feeds parasites. The liver starts to cleanse usually after a few colonics. Now you are on your way to super natural health. You can expect to see a dramatic flattening of your stomach. Many people will lose between 5-to-20 pounds just from a series of colonics alone! Also, you will drastically reduce bloating, gas, food cravings, and constipation—not to mention improved digestion, increased energy and mental clarity, and a better absorption of nutrients and an overall health improvement.

Probiotics

During your series of colonics, you will want to take probiotics to ensure healthy digestive conditions and a healthy bacterial flora as you rid yourself of the "bad stuff." Probiotics will put into your system friendly bacteria that will trigger your metabolism, improve digestion, and help with the cleansing process during colonics. I recommend taking them right after your colonic and then the following 3 days on an empty stomach following your colonic.

During your colonic series you will also want to alkanize your body with lots of greens and green-leafy vegetable juices. With colonics, chlorophyll and chlorella help to speed up the detox process pulling out harmful toxins from the body such as heavy metals, mercury, and foreign chemicals. To remineralize your body you can buy encapsulated organic wild bluegreen algae, chlorella, and organic spirulina. You can find these and other supplements at superhealthvitamins.com.

Liver

Once the liver detoxifies, which is one of your primary objectives, all the other organs start to follow. The liver detoxifies even more quickly when fasting on juice or fresh spring water as it is less overloaded with excess toxins. Lots of cooked animal foods and cooked fried foods on a consistent basis without the balance of raw foods are difficult for the body to metabolize and detoxify. By reducing or eliminating animal and fried foods during fasting, you are really helping your body with its goal of flushing out all the old waste matter so you can start to nourish it with real superfoods. Most people have a clogged or sluggish liver. When this starts to occur, your metabolism slows down as fat stores increase, digestion slows down, appetites increase, and food cravings increase. When this occurs, your body's immune system and liver get overloaded, causing symptoms and diseases over time.

When you cleanse your liver, because it is no longer overtaxed, every organ in your body starts to function more efficiently. The result is you will have more energy, less depression, increased metabolism, less over-eating, and an overall sense of well-being. Only do a liver cleanse after you have done a series of colonics. Then your body starts to rebuild.

An unhealthy body will suddenly become changed into a new healthy body through detox. Eating living foods will help with mental clarity and a positive outlook—going from a natural to a supernatural being. Colonics will start to cleanse your liver, but it is also helpful to do a separate liver cleanse after a series of colonics.

Candida Cleanse

Most people on western diets have some level of Candida and yeast overgrowth. These also cause bloating, constipation, poor digestion, gas, hormonal imbalances, tiredness and other ailments. A Candida cleanse is excellent for getting rid of live Candida organisms that live inside of your gut that feed on your toxins as well as the yeast. You can simply take Candida cleanse tablets every night for 1 or 2 months even during colonics. You will, of course, have to refrain from most sweets and sweet fruits during this time as they often feed on sugary foods. If you do not address Candida, your food cravings will continue.

These are the main cleanses you should start with, but the most important to start with is the colonics that will take you into a new dimension of health even after your first series and even your first few colonics.

Infrared Sauna: Skin Cleaning

This is another fantastic way to cleanse other organs of your body at the same time. The skin is the largest organ of your body. When you start cleansing more frequently, it will come out of your skin. One of the best ways to speed up the cleansing process is to allow your skin to sweat out the toxins. Saunas are the best way to do this—especially infrared saunas. Sweating in a sauna increases metabolism releasing accumulated toxins while also stimulating the release of fat cells. Any sauna will help of course, but infrared saunas go much deeper—a cellular level of cleansing. Sweating for 20-to-30 minutes a day using a sauna is highly recommended and will increase weight loss and the elimination of toxins.

Your skin, being the largest organ in one's body, naturally accumulates toxins and waste as much as anything else even while showering with normal chlorinated city water. Sweating in a sauna helps to stimulate the release of accumulated toxins, which in turn increases your metabolism, reduces your appetite and increases metabolic rate. Sweating for 20 to 30 minutes a day will have amazing health benefits, increase weight loss and eliminate toxins.

Infrared saunas penetrate much deeper on the cellular level than conventional saunas and take less time. The deep heat penetration of infrared saunas removes not only toxins but alcohol, nicotine, and metals; they help cure chronic fatigue, promote muscle growth, and reduce cellulite. Also, you lose more calories, (up to 600 calories or more) sitting in this type of sauna for 30 minutes than you would running for the same amount of time. It's great because if you don't always have time to exercise, you can sit in one of these and read a book or listen to a CD and get the same benefits as running or cardio in the same amount of time. Infrared saunas also help to significantly de-stress you.

Infrared saunas help with blood circulation leaving you more beautiful, youthful, and with glowing skin—a great help in reducing acne and even scars. Many people have found pain relief for arthritis, back pain, muscle spasms, and headaches from infrared saunas. Athletes use them to quickly recover from sprains, arthritis, muscle spasms, and back pain as the deep heat penetrates much deeper than a normal sauna.

Another thing infrared saunas do is raise oxygenation and remove radioactive residues. They also are good for chronic infections and have been found to be helpful to cancer patients. Infrared saunas require less energy and heat much faster than traditional saunas. They help patients suffering from varicose veins, metal implants, hypertension, and diabetes where conventional saunas do not achieve these same results.

To increase the benefits of infrared sauna use, you can use a dry brush and brush off the skin. This helps remove the toxins after your session before showering and stimulates circulation. Skin brushing daily during your cleanse is also beneficial. Vigorously brush your skin before or during your shower or bath. Because the skin is the largest organ in your body, brushing has significant benefits.

Because of their amazing health benefits now becoming known to more people, infrared saunas are more affordable than ever. You can now purchase very portable, lightweight infrared saunas for under $2,000. Whether you live in an apartment, mobile home, or large house, far infrared saunas are designed to be stored in any apartment or housing situation—even outdoors. I use one regularly now after I experienced their amazing benefits. This is one investment in your health that you can't afford to overlook.

Massage

While doing a series of colon and other cleanses getting massages during this time will greatly aid in pushing the toxins and lactic acid out of your system rapidly and increase circulation. Massage reduces stiffness. The best type of massages for stiffness that I recommend are deep tissue and Thai massage, but there are other types as well that could be beneficial.

Cardiovascular Workout

During your cleanse you will want to exercise at least three times a week with some sort of cardiovascular workout. Exercising during your cleanse will help you to cleanse much faster through sweating and improving your blood circulation by elevating your heart rate. Exercise also affects your hormones and body chemistry increasing your overall sense of wellbeing giving you more mental and emotional clarity and higher self-esteem. It's also a great stress reliever and relaxes you. One of the best things you can do daily for sure is to walk for 1 hour a day or as much as you can—building up to 1 hour. By doing this, every cell in your body starts to get cleansed and it keeps your heart, blood, and many other organs clean. It's best to walk outdoors. Getting fresh air affects your body immensely. Also, you feel more grounded when walking outdoors as the earth is always moving and rotating, keeping you grounded when walking on the earth itself. The opposite is true, for example, when you are in a car or airplane all the time or on long trips. Once you get out you feel unbalanced and unconnected. Walking outdoors keeps you grounded as the human body was made to walk.

Water

You need to drink lots of water throughout the day when cleansing. This will help in pushing the toxins through your system rapidly as you are detoxing and cleansing on many levels simultaneously. Staying hydrated will also give you more energy. Your body is made primarily of water. You want to use the best water possible. Spring water or filtered water are the best. If you can get a water filter for your home that is even better as you will eliminate the harmful chlorine and chemicals that enter your bloodstream every time you take a shower. Also you will then have an unlimited supply of good drinking water.

Rebounding

One of the great benefits of rebounding is that it cleanses your lymphatic system.

Rebounding flushes the lymph—the toxic substances that the body is always rounding up from its normal processes, such as food wastes and environmental pollutants—before they can form new waste by-products. Dr. Walker sums it up: "[During rebounding] arterial blood enters the capillaries in order to furnish the cells with fresh tissue fluid containing food and oxygen. The bouncing motion moves and recycles the lymph and the entire blood supply through the circulatory system many times during the course of the rebounding session." The feature of rebounding that sets it apart from all other exercises is that half of the time you do it you are not opposing gravity! When you are bounced upward by the springs and mat of the quality rebounder, your body is not being pulled by gravity. Because of this action, each cell in the body and brain receives a positive stress. And the joy of it is that you don't have to exert yourself to get these benefits. The eldest of the elderly, the handicapped and the arthritic can do this, by doing a very gentle, 2-to-3-minute "health bounce."

What is the "health bounce"?

The lymphatic system, as Dr. Morton Walker refers to it in his book *Jumping for Health*, is the "metabolic garbage can of the body. It rids you of toxins, such as dead and cancerous cells, nitrogenous wastes, fat, infectious viruses, heavy metals, and other material cast off by the cells." The lymphatic fluid is a clear liquid that contains the body's T- and B-cells, or cells that help the immune system ward off disease. When you rebound, you help your cells metabolize, cleanse, and renew, and you help your lymph system to pump and drain the body's waste. The cardiovascular hydraulics benefit too. Linda Brooks, author of *Rebounding for Health* writes, "Lymph is moved like a hydraulic pressure system. The lymph tubes are filled with one-way valves that only open up, or allow drainage toward the center of the body. When pressure below the valve is greater than above (as when you are moving downward on the rebounder), the valves are forced open so the fluid can flow." There are about three ways for the lymph system to "pump" and cleanse: exercise, which helps muscular contraction; massage (via movement) of the musculature or tissues. It serves to get it to pump back into the pulmonary circulation; and gravitational pressure with its resultant internal massage. Rebounding, remarkably, provides all three ways of removing waste from cells.

Medical researchers agree that aside from poor nutrition, the primary cause of fatigue, disease, cell degeneration, and premature aging is poor circulation to and from the tissues of the body. Rebounding gives you the most efficient forms of tissue oxygenation and blood circulation. Rebounding will help you to stimulate lymphatic circulation, which means the broken down products of fat metabolism as well as toxins can drain out of your body through your liver and spleen. It can also help you rebuild cells that are stronger, healthier, more oxygen-enriched and more resilient disease fighters.

Chapter 2

Super Natural Food

"It's funny about life: if you refuse to accept anything but the very best you will very often get it."
—William Somerset Maugham

There is a lot of truth to *You are what you eat!* Many of the ancients lived off of the food that grew off the earth untouched by modern day ills and seemed to have supernatural bodies and lifestyles. Contemporary food has deprived most people today of this euphoric feeling of health creating multitudes of new sicknesses never heard of before.

What you eat will totally determine your quality of life on earth, your mental and emotional state as well as your spiritual state depending on which way you go about it. Your body is a tool that needs to be harnessed to allow you to achieve your maximum potential in every area of your life.

A correct diet that includes superfood intake gives you a major edge over most people in the modern world. When you give your body superfoods, they propel your mind, body, emotions, and spiritual life to new highs that you never could have achieved.

When people fast for a season, they report having euphoric feelings, clear minds and better concentration. They are able to connect to the spiritual world so much easier. They also receive fresh creative inspiration, ideas, and direction. This is because they are temporarily cleansing themselves from most of the harmful things in our food today. Nothing bad is coming in and they are detoxing during their fast and resurrecting their spiritual senses. Their energy is not being used to digest food that overloads all the organs, but instead connects them to higher planes of thinking, feeling, and being. Once these blockages are removed, people's minds unclog allowing them to think more creatively, emotions get more into balance, and they feel physically well—like they can soar like an eagle during their fast.

Imagine having that same kind of feeling every day even without fasting but eating in such a way that you are always on a "high" because of changing what you eat and your lifestyle. You would be going from a natural to a supernatural being in no time—achieving your lifelong goals and dreams much easier because your mind, body, will, emotions, and spirit would all be congruently connected toward your goals, each enabling the other.

ENERGY FIELDS

People often like to go camping, connect with nature, swim in the ocean, and go on nature hikes. You will notice that when you are on a vacation in a nature setting you feel more relaxed and de-stressed. You get fresh insights and inspiration. One of the reasons is that the energy field of nature, trees, rocks, and unspoiled forests carry a much higher energy frequency than being in the downtown area of an inner city, where most everything is manmade and polluted. Most artists like to be in natural surroundings in the mountains or on the beach as they seem to tap into a higher level of creativity. The closer you get to natural raw creation, the closer you get to the Creator where you start to draw fresh creative abilities and thoughts that you would not otherwise receive. Most people living in stressful city environments consume less than nutritious dead foods and feel like they are in "survival mode"—trying to fight the traffic to get home only to watch toxic programs that increase stress and cortisone levels.

The foods you eat also carry certain energy fields. Some food carry high frequency energy fields and other have much lower levels. The higher the energy field of the foods you eat, the healthier you will be. Some foods are considered "dead food" which carry almost no energy but zap your energy and health.

The highest energy-rich superfoods are uncooked raw plant foods. They are the most perfect food for human consumption. The reason is that the plants derive their energy directly from the sun. When you eat them, that energy is directly ingested into your system. Superfoods cleanse, energize, and come out of your system rapidly. The cleaner your body is, the more you will radiate from a natural to a supernatural being that people will notice and be changed by. When you eat only cooked food, most of the enzymes and superfood nutrients have been destroyed, giving you much less nutrition It often takes more cooked food to get that full feeling—they have much less nutrients—and also contribute to weight gain and toxins. The ideal goal would be to eat at least 80 percent raw to detox and start on your journey to super natural health.

A toxic life and environment destroys your energy, joy, and outlook. It dulls your senses and supernatural abilities degenerating you into much less than you were created to be. A toxic life causes you to live in a duller survival state as opposed to a creative supercharged "excited about life" state of mind. Once you change your food intake, your dormant abilities start to resurface and suddenly you are happy, positive, and feel great—able to live your life to its fullest in every area—opening up your untapped genius!

Raw Plant Food—Super Natural Food

Raw plant foods are the ultimate source of pure energy and pure healing foods that you need to eat daily. The quicker you eat food in its rawest natural form, the quicker you will possess incredible energy, health, vitality and strength as your entire being will be transformed.

Edible plants are a powerhouse of live, raw, instantly absorbed energy fields. They receive energy directly from sunlight and fresh air; you in turn ingest powerful energy fields of life. Your energy vibrations rise. On the other hand, when you eat processed food with low or negative raw energy, your entire body is thrown off. Food that is synthetic, refined, or processed totally depletes the body of energy, strength, and health—a slow death. Slowly but surely, this type of lifestyle eating robs you of the health, joy, and freedom spiraling your body toward death much faster.

The idea is to try and consume as much raw food as you can. Most people can start off at least eating 50 percent raw foods and then gradually increasing this to 80 percent raw plant foods and 20 percent cooked foods. When you eat only cooked food you destroy the enzymes that help to break down that food. The more enzymes you get throughout the day from raw foods, the faster it flushes toxins and junk out of your body continually cleansing, healing, and energizing you, instead of adding to the problem of clogging your system.

Different foods carry different levels of energy fields. The higher the food energy, the better it is for you. Anything that alters the food would lower the energy frequency such as microwaving, canning, freezing, pesticides, and cooking. Frozen food, for example, destroys anywhere from 30 percent to 60 percent of the enzymes in the food. But it still is better and less damaging than cooked food. The more natural you go, the better. Everyone has to start somewhere and knowing the different levels of natural to unnatural food really helps in transitioning.

HIGHEST ENERGY FOOD

Eating fresh raw organic vegetables and organic sun-ripened, raw fresh fruit are on the top of the list of highest energy foods that will take you from natural to super natural in no time. The more raw green vegetables and raw fruit you eat the better. Especially those that are organic—untouched by pesticides.

MEDIUM ENERGY FOOD

Other foods that are still higher energy than most cooked foods but not as high-energy as raw plants and fruits would be things like some cooked vegetables, raw organic goat milk and cheese, raw organic nuts and seeds, and raw sprouted grains. These would be considered medium energy foods.

LOWER ENERGY FOOD

(But still totally acceptable as you transition)

Some of the lower energy foods but still totally acceptable during transition for the long term combined with high energy foods would be free-range organic eggs, organic wild fish (for example, wild salmon which is much higher energy than beef or chicken and digests much quicker), raw cow milk, and raw cold pressed oils. As you are transitioning from dead foods to higher energy foods, you will most likely be eating a variety of high, middle, and low-energy foods.

NEUTRAL FOODS DURING TRANSITION

Neutral foods are not ideal foods on a daily basis but as you are transitioning toward your goal, they will help to make the transition from destructive foods into a more healthy lifestyle.

Some of these foods could be free-range, grass-fed, and organic meats, whole-grain products, non-raw organic cheeses
(but not as great as raw goat cheese).

These are examples but again the idea is to try and consume
for the most part raw plants and fruits as much as possible or as
closest to 50 percent, then 80 percent as you can.

Dead and Destructive Foods

These are foods that you should stop eating right away if you are
to start on this path of total health. For starters, this would be
pasteurized dairy products of any kind including regular pasteurized milk, yogurt, and cheese. (Raw is fine.) The reason is that the
pasteurization process has already destroyed all the enzymes and
nutrients in the dairy product leaving nothing but digestion and
other complications. Other destructive foods, starting with the
most to the least detrimental to eliminate would be most animal
fleshes that are not wild, organic and/or grass-fed like pork, cow
meat (beef), chicken, lamb, game, and farm-raised fish (wild fish
is the best choice).

These foods are filled with hormones and steroids that stay
in the meats and in your bloodstream. Pork, for example, is the
worst because it is literally a meat that clogs up your arteries more
than any other meat and has the highest amount of parasites. It is
a food that was not necessarily designed for human consumption
and doctors often tell people to stop eating pork when things get
clogged up. Beef, chicken, and most mainstream meats that are
not organic are so filled with hormones and other chemicals that
they slow you down and reverse the healing processes in your
body. These also take the longest to digest and eliminate from
your system. Any food that stays long in your system tires you
out the most and has the highest probability of causing sickness.
(Remember the last time you had that big non-organic late-night
steak dinner, you felt pretty sleepy and drowsy shortly after.)

Whatever food that does not get digested quickly will stay in your colon building up fecal matter and start to putrefy along the walls of your intestines causing colon and other problems in the future. Everything in your body starts to slow down—blocking the absorption of nutrients—causing many other problems over the years. You don't have to be a vegetarian but if you do eat meat like wild fish, as long as you stay on the high-energy foods at the same time, you will be doing so much better than most of the population. Try and cut out the rest of the meats as much as possible but go at your own pace daily adding more high energy food while slowly but surely (or quickly) eliminating destructive food.

Juicing and Blending
The secret to tapping into all the raw power of food.

Fresh raw organic vegetables and fruits that have just been juiced or blended are the most concentrated, edible, nutrients filled with energy that exist!

When you use a juicer or blender, liquid supernatural energy bypasses chewing and shoots nutrients and raw energy straight into your bloodstream giving you a euphoric high—raw food in liquid form.

Juicing and blending your raw food smoothies not only tastes incredibly good but is the fastest way of going from natural to supernatural eating. It also tastes so good. All you need to do is to mix some fruit with the raw plants and the taste and sensation is out of this world. Also you are hydrating and oxygenating your cells every time you liquefy your fresh raw veggies and fruits.

What I like to do upon waking up is to make a liquid super-food drink—this is the first substance to hit my body causing a supernatural energy burst before doing or eating anything else. I often like to throw in some spinach, kale, celery, and two apples along with either water or coconut water for added flavor. In a couple of seconds you have liquid energy ready to consume! You are on your way to sensations of pure energetic bliss! Just stick to it and make it a lifestyle as opposed to a temporary diet. (Going back to dead foods once you are on high super natural energy diets will often make you depressed as you will see the major difference and wonder how you went this long eating the way you did.)

Blenders vs. Juicers

People use juicers because they feel they will get more nutrients in their diets this way. Juicers are different than blenders in that they use an extractor to extract only the juice of fruits and vegetables while removing the pulp and the fiber. The theory is that, by removing the fiber, your body can easily absorb much higher levels of nutrients directly into the bloodstream.

The only problem with this is if you are juicing, for example, sweet fruits and carrots, then the high sugar content will cause a spike to your blood since the fiber has been removed that would have otherwise balanced out the sugar. Nature intended for the whole food to be eaten. Juicing works best if you are using dark green leafy vegetables. In this way, you can maximize the nutrients you receive straight to your blood without a spike in your sugar.

Because juicing removes fiber, which is often the most nutritious part of a food, people can get constipated if you do a lot of juicing as you are often not getting enough fiber in your diet.

An example: The white skin of oranges is packed with phytonutrients that you really need. It is actually better to eat a raw organic fruit than to mix it when it comes to fruits. Juice goes down quickly, is digested quickly, and is absorbed into the bloodstream quickly. As a result, you become hungrier more quickly. Since smoothies contain fiber, you will feel full longer. High-fiber content means it will take longer to digest, meaning you won't become hungry as quickly. Further, since juicing requires many fruits and vegetables, the juice—ounce for ounce—is **higher in calories and sugar** than a smoothie made in a blender. I have gone through many blenders and the best one that lasts the longest hands-down is the Vita-Mix. It handles the largest amount of food as it's much larger than other blenders and is the most sturdy of blenders as it can even liquefy the pit of an avocado.

The great thing about blending is that you get the entire fruit or vegetable as if you chewed it. This way all the nutrients are in the food, including the fiber. It's the ultimate tool to make quick, delicious meals. Making raw super-smoothies with your blender is also so tasty. A juicer is much more time-consuming and takes much more time to clean.

It is easier to pack in more nutrients with a blender than with just eating a salad, and you get it faster into your system as the blender has done the work of chewing the food down to a liquid form. It saves you time in eating. If you are in a hurry, the time it would take you to make a huge organic salad and eat it could easily take you an hour. But just throw your salad in the blender like spinach, kale, avocado, and maybe and apple or two and you can drink it quickly and be on your way, getting all the same raw nutrients and usually much more than eating and also much quicker absorption into your system!

If you have the time and want to get the most of out both juicing and blending, then the best way is to juice your vegetables then pour the juice into a blender and add fruits into the blender so that you keep the fiber content. That way you have the best of both worlds. As far as vegetables go, juicing is very beneficial. Many who are sick have used it to heal very quickly. Veggies that are blended usually take about 2 hours to be absorbed and digested, but when juiced take only 30 minutes to be digested. So if you combine both juicer and blender, juicing for vegetables and blending for fruits, and mix them together you get the best of both worlds. But believe me, if you don't have the time and are starting out, you still will get major benefits from putting both raw veggies and a little fruit in the blender compared with not doing anything at all, and your food will be much easier to absorb. When blending, you are still getting the whole food as if you chewed it as nature intended.

WHY ORGANIC?

Some people say that it is too costly to buy organic. Actually, it is more costly not to eat organic given the lower nutritional value of most foods and the sicknesses, diseases and health care costs it would take to try and treat most modern sicknesses that most doctors don't really cure but control with harmful drugs. Spending the extra money is totally worth it and will never be a loss as you will start to reap the benefits immediately. Just think of it as investing in your own health care so you don't have to be operated or "experimented" on with pharmaceutical drugs later on.

Organic foods, for one, are in their raw natural state. They are not sprayed with pesticides, chemicals, fungicides, and other harmful things. Organically grown food also has much lower quantities of toxic trace minerals like lead, mercury, and aluminum.

Studies have shown that organic food contains way more iron, potassium, magnesium, and calcium than conventional crops. Most studies show organic food having up to 10 times the mineral content of conventional foods. You really get more nutrition for your money.

What is amazing is that you feel full faster on a smaller portion of raw organic food than you do with processed foods. I remember going to get a hamburger at a fast-food place and I could eat so many of those hamburgers. The reason is that your body is not getting the nutrients it needs so it continues to tell you that you are still hungry when in reality that food is just being stored—contributing to weight gain and stuck in your gut confused as to where it goes in the body as it is not natural. All the while you keep eating, thinking you are still hungry. On the other hand, I can eat an organic salad with lettuce, avocado, and other fresh vegetables and it usually fills me up in one serving because my body is getting the nutrients and the healthy fats it needs—telling me that I am full. For example, organic spinach contains 64 to 78 percent more vitamin C than non-organic.

Other tests done showed that organically grown pears have 2-to-3 times more chromium, iodine, manganese, molybdenum, silicon, and zinc. Organic potatoes have 2-to-3 times more boron, selenium, silicon, strontium, and sulfur and 60 percent more zinc. Organic corn has 20 times more calcium and manganese, and 2-to-5 times more copper, magnesium, molybdenum, selenium, and zinc than non-organic. Organic wheat has, for example, 13 times more selenium than commercial wheat and with twice the calcium.

EASY IN EASY OUT FOODS

Foods that digest quickly are the best. Once you have started a cleanse with a combination of colonics and other cleanses it would be crazy to go back to your normal diet, only to get clogged up again. What you need to do now is to eat more raw organic food. Raw plants and raw fruits are the easiest foods to digest—they do not stay in your system but work to get in and get the heck out as fast as possible.

Let's say you are just starting to go from an unhealthy low-energy diet to a high-energy diet and you are somewhere in between. You just ordered a steak and potatoes meal wondering what will happen. Well that steak will spend about 8-to-12 hours in your stomach taking the entire night to digest, sapping your body of vital energy needed to cleanse organs like your liver. While you sleep, your liver is being clogged up working overtime trying to compensate the entire time you are sleeping after the meal. You wake up feeling tired and groggy because your body did not really rest but tried playing catch up—digesting all night. On the other hand, if you ate a raw salad with that steak, as bad for you as the steak was, the time in your stomach would be reduced to only 4 or 5 hours just from adding raw salad. This alone would greatly reduce your bloating, weight gain, and clogging of your system. Often, when you think you are craving meat, you are actually craving healthy fats like avocado. Try making an avocado salad and notice how your meat cravings drastically diminish especially in the evening.

You see where I am going with this. Any changes you start to make with the goal of going between 50 percent up to at least 80 percent raw will have a total change on your life and health! Of course the better meal would be the wild salmon with the salad as that would digest much faster than the steak if you are just beginning.

Imagine if you did not eat meat at night at all right before bedtime as most weight is gained from whatever you eat after 6 p.m. Imagine the energy you would have upon awaking only to consume a raw organic vegetable and fruit juice. The more alkalized and raw the food you eat, the more it will prevent waste matter building up, keeping you full of health, vitality, and energy!

As your body becomes cleansed, all that extra energy used to deal with digesting a clogged system will be unleashed. As your body is more rested, you start to tap into the creative side of your brain with fresh ideas that before you could not clearly focus on as your thoughts were more clouded. You start to become a receiver of ideas, inventions, and projects that were there all along but you could not grasp them until you went from natural to super natural health.

Energy Fields

Today, research has been done to demonstrate that food, objects, and people have varying levels of energy. Einstein's theory of relativity, $E = mc^2$ is still a fact today. Energy is matter. Everything you see consisting of matter is made up of energy. Some foods have higher energy fields than others. Those that are raw and organic emanate higher energy fields as their energy has not been destroyed or altered by unnatural means. When you eat these high-energy foods, you turn into a high-energy person. Other things that increase or decrease your healthy energy field is what you think about and your attitude, which we will cover later. Researchers have come up with a way to actually photograph the energy levels of objects including food. In one photo a fruit that is uncooked looks like a supernova sun exploding with brilliant light. In the next photo, the same fruit cooked has almost no light coming out of it compared with the first photo and it looks somewhat deformed. It is really true that you are what you eat. Are you planning on being a high-energy person? If so, read on and enjoy a new beginning!

Chapter 3

Weight Loss

"Nothing tastes as good as being thin feels."
—Anonymous

Weight loss seems to be an obsession these days. Ads for miracle weight loss cures are all over the place. The problem is that most of these cures do not work and once the weight is lost it comes right back because the cures do not address the deeper issues of what causes weight gain. Once you tackle that issue, then you not only lose weight, you can easily keep it off.

What you will learn here is not a diet but a lifestyle. The more of these things that you incorporate in your daily life the faster the results. Try to incorporate these strategies into your lifestyle daily by adding at least one or two of these things until they become a habit.

As a nutrition coach, motivational speaker, researcher, life coach and health enthusiast and after years of research and experimentation, using these principles and strategies myself, I have seen amazing results both personally and in other people's lives. Get ready to go from natural to super natural health while experiencing weight loss and recover your life, joy, and energy once again!

HINDRANCES TO WEIGHT LOSS

Before I share with you secrets to losing weight, I need to address first what causes the weight gain and what not to do. As you know from Chapter 1, food that is not organic sold in most stores, fast-food places, and chain restaurants is loaded with chemicals, toxins, and processed junk that totally clog you up and cause you to get addicted. The false advertising seducing millions to eat totally non-nourishing addictive foods is a great contributor to this epidemic of overweight problems. Many things today have caused people's metabolism to slow down. Our metabolisms need to be revved back up naturally. Here are some of the main causes of weight gain that if avoided will start to reverse this problem.

1. **Clogged Colon:** Your colon gets clogged by dehydration (lack of water), lack of fiber, lack of walking and exercise, lack of enzymes in your food, pharmaceutical prescription and non-prescription drugs. Cleansing your colon is an absolute must! **If you do not have three bowel movements daily, then you have a clogged colon.** From autopsies, doctors have found as much as 30 pounds of undigested putrefied fecal matter in human colons that contributed to their death. If ignored, your metabolism will continue to slow down, your hunger pains will be higher and higher as your body will signal that it's not getting enough nutrients causing you to overeat. Your digestion will always be slow and your stomach will stay bloated— never flat as it was meant to be. I recommend starting with a colon cleanse, followed by liver and Candida cleanses. Once the colon is cleansed, it will start to cleanse the liver and then an additional liver cleanse can be added later depending on how clogged you are.

2. **Clogged liver:** Almost everyone who is overweight that has ever been tested is found to have a sluggish clogged liver. Many things cause one's liver to be clogged. Some of the

main culprits are a clogged colon, trans fats, prescription, and non-prescription drugs, Candida yeast overgrowth, artificial sweeteners, non-organic toxic foods, and many other things. When your liver is clogged, your body starts to rapidly store high levels of body fat. Metabolism always slows down when the liver is clogged greatly contributing to weight gain. (Doing the cleanses in Chapter 1 will help you unclog your liver as you will start to drop pounds from the cleanses alone and speed up weight loss there after.)

3. **Candida:** Most people in the western world or on western diets have some form of Candida. Candida causes food cravings for things like bread, pasta, cheese, sweets/sugar etc. Candida blocks your colon slowing down metabolism and digestion. It causes gas, bloating, and a stomach that is never flat. Once you take your first antibiotic, it starts to destroy your good bacteria allowing for bad bacteria like Candida yeast to start growing at abnormal rates. Eventually if not corrected through a Candida cleanse it turns into a fungus that spreads throughout your entire body system. (Once you have done a colon and liver cleanse the next cleanse I recommend is a Candida cleanse. You will lose pounds just by doing this cleanse with greater health benefits.) The goal is not just weight loss but total health with weight loss that stays off because you are addressing the causes instead of just getting a temporary result.

4. **Parasites:** If you are overweight, I can guarantee you have parasites. Parasites are caused by a clogged colon, liver, Candida, heavy metal toxicity, and lack of nutrients among other things.

5. **Enzyme deficient:** Food that is not organic or has been pasteurized or cooked (anything heated over 180 degrees for 30 minutes) has no enzymes. Most people even when eating vegetables cook them and never get the enzymes or the full nutrients they need. (There are a few exceptions with some

veggies that are better slightly cooked/steamed but that is the exception not the rule). Without enough enzymes you will always have trouble digesting food, low metabolism, gas, constipation, and bloating. A lifestyle change of eating more raw foods and eating fresh raw salads with any of your cooked food and especially juicing your raw veggies will help to correct a deficiency of enzymes in your diet. Everything will then be easily digested and metabolized. As you start your diet, a good idea would be to add some enzyme tablets to your meals. Overweight people are hindered in their ability to create enough enzymes to digest their food properly due to highly refined foods, pasteurized foods, clogged liver and colon, prescription, and non-prescription drugs. At least, at the beginning of your journey you should take some supplemental enzymes with each meal to get your body back to normal.

6. **Stress:** If you are stressed on an ongoing basis, you will store fat. There are things you can do to relieve stress no matter what your job description or lifestyle is at present, which we will cover later on in the book. Overexposure to cell phones, TV, electronic devices, and other currents going through your system also stress your body and entire system.

7. **Water deficient:** Most people do not consume enough water and are dehydrated. Much of the liquids they do consume like sodas and most popular caffeine drinks lead to more dehydration. Without pure drinking water your cells cannot properly hydrate, which contributes to a slower metabolism. Those who drink tap water clog their system with lots of phosphorous, chlorine, heavy metals, and toxins among other things. You need fresh water.

8. **Food additives:** If you are not eating organic food all the time then you are consuming pesticides, chemical fertilizers, herbicides, thousands of artificial chemicals and antibiotics especially if you live in North America. Many nations

are copying this western diet and catching up quick to U.S. obesity levels.

9. **Fast-food Restaurants:** Every single fast-food restaurant and national or regional chain restaurant (especially in westernized nations) should be avoided as you start to achieve supernatural health and weight loss. Their foods are generally loaded with trans fats, high processed sugars and fructose corn syrup, MSG, artificial corn sweeteners, and nitrates. Meats and dairy from fast food places and many national chain restaurants are always full of growth hormones, antibiotics, and drugs. Often the food is microwaved. These foods often have no fiber and are highly processed. Such foods are designed by companies to ensure big profits; they create foods that increase hunger and cause you to be addicted in every way. These foods lead to depression and make you gain weight.

10. **Sodas and carbonated drinks:** Carbonated drinks and sodas block calcium absorption, which lowers metabolism and causes nutritional deficiencies. Sodas loaded with sugar are the worst offenders—the diet drinks are actually worse.

11. **Sugar/Sweeteners:** When your body is overloaded with sugars and desserts, high fructose corn syrup, and other sweeteners, weight gain occurs fast. Sodas including diet sodas (diet sodas cause cancer because of the replacement sweeteners they use) have so much sugar in one can that your system goes into shock and overloads—storing up fast. High amounts of fat are stored and insulin levels get out of whack. Even artificial sweeteners—aspartame, sucralose and popular ones such as Splenda and NutraSweet—will slow your metabolism.

12. **Lack of Sleep:** Studies have proven that less than 7 hours of sleep per night leads to obesity. (The best time to sleep is around 10 p.m. or earlier as your liver starts to detox and cleanses every night between 10 p.m. and 2 a.m. when in

deep sleep.) Lack of sleep and inconsistent sleep times on a regular basis hinder the cleansing process—slowing down metabolism.

13. **Lack of Exercise:** Poor circulation causes our metabolism to slow down. Circulation problems can be due to clogged arteries caused by poor nutrition with lots of trans fats, pasteurized dairy products, chlorine in your water, Candida, heavy metals and so on. Lack of exercise contributes to poor circulation. The human body was made to walk. This is the most basic but effective exercise to improve circulation. In most countries people walk a minimum of 5 miles a day or more. In America for instance, the average person walks less than a tenth of a mile daily! When you walk you get everything in your system circulating and cleansing out the cells rejuvenates your entire system.

14. **Sunlight deficient:** When you are out in the sun it activates your metabolism to speed up. It also reduces stress; sunshine has been proven to greatly diminish depression.

15. **Lack of Sweating/Perspiration:** The largest organ of your body is your skin. It is supposed to eliminate the toxins from your body on a regular basis. A lack of sweating clogs your lymphatic system and slows metabolism. As much as people love air-conditioning, we need to also sweat to be healthy and lose weight and toxins. This is another modern-world lifestyle deficiency. It has been proven that air conditioning and a lack of regular sunlight lower metabolism.

16. **Weak muscle mass:** If you don't maintain normal muscle mass through certain exercises or work, your metabolism will be slower. When you increase muscle mass, your metabolism speeds up. If you increase muscle through exercise, this helps burn fat and increase metabolism all the time—even while you sleep.

These are just some of the things that contribute to weight gain that you want to keep in mind. When your metabolism is slow it keeps you tired, groggy, lethargic and you start to lack passion and creativity. Once you start to make certain simple adjustments and changes, you will be amazed at the weight you lose as you continue your journey from a natural to a super natural life.

Lose Weight Now

The following items, if adapted, will cause you to increase your metabolism, burn fat and lose weight. The more of these things you do on a regular daily basis, the more weight you will lose while increasing in health. I put these in the order of priority and importance.

Drink Water: Drink a large glass of water as soon as you wake up before doing anything else. Drink spring water or filtered water by reverse osmosis. People who are overweight are always dehydrated, whether they know it or not. Drink lots of it throughout the day to flush out your system (Never drink tap water as it will clog you as it has tons of fluoride, chlorine, and other harmful chemicals.) If you drink bottled water, try to buy glass bottles as opposed to plastic bottles because the plastic often leaks into the water over time and is known to add unhealthy estrogen into your system.

Do Cardio Exercise: I suggest walking, running, or even swimming as fast and as brisk as you can for about 15-to-20 minutes before breakfast and before lunch. When you wake up, your body is in a semi fasted state and will start to burn fat right away when you exercise before breakfast. Then later in the day walk for at least 1 hour outside non-stop or at least work up to that goal. (Maybe start with 30 minutes, then 40, then 1 hour.) For those in better athletic shape, running will increase your weight loss. But as a rule of thumb make it your goal to at least simply walk for 1 hour a day but knowing that any amount you can do daily will only increase your weight loss. (This can be separate from or in place of the brisk walking or cardio like swimming before breakfast and lunch.)

Do Rebounding: Rebounding also is a great addition to walking. It stimulates the lymphatic system, releases helpful endorphins and other hormones and is the only exercise in the world that stimulates and exercises every single cell in your entire body all at the same time—releasing toxins, improving circulation, increasing muscle tone, flexibility, and oxygenating the blood. You can just set up a rebounder in front of your TV or in your office and simply bounce for 5 or 10 minutes once or twice a day. By doing this, you will notice super natural physical, emotional, and mental health benefits—a great aid in weight loss. I use one practically every day when at home.

Do a Colonics Cleanse: Before you put it off why not right now make an appointment with a licensed colon therapist to get your health and weight loss goals activated! Do a series anywhere from 6-to-15 colonics during a 30-day period. Your therapist during the first few sessions will know how many you need depending on how fast you cleanse and how clogged up you are. To speed up the colon being cleansed you can start to take a colon cleanse product in tablet form during your series of colonics or anytime before or after. Once you finish your series, do a liver and Candida cleanse.

Eat Fat-busting Fruits/Veggies: Eat at least two organic apples daily as they are a great fiber, they fill you up fast—reducing appetite and help in cleansing the liver, gallbladder, and colon.

Try to eat two grapefruits a day as the enzymes in grapefruits are high and they burn and release fat stores as well as cleanse all the vital organs. Eat also at least one organic avocado a day either with a salad or alone. These have the healthy fats that help you lose weight and give you a sense of being full. Drink 2 teaspoons a day of extra virgin raw coconut oil as it also really helps release fat cells, digestion, speed metabolism—among other things. Adding 1 tablespoon of raw organic apple cider vinegar also stimulates the release of stored fat cells, cleanses, and speeds up metabolism.

Eat Fiber: Increasing dietary fiber will drastically accelerate weight loss, improve digestion, clean out toxins, help turn back years of eating refined processed foods, relieve constipation, reduce appetite and so on. Taking extra fiber during the first phase of your journey will be a big help.

Drink Teas: The best tea for giving natural energy and speeding up metabolism is green tea and Yerba Mate. Yerba Mate is my favorite as it increases energy but without the jitters that normal coffee gives you and without the crash feeling afterward. It stimulates the release of fat cells and reduces appetite. Drink at least 1 cup a day of both Yerba Mate and Green Tea. I like to mix mine together.

Eat 100 Percent Organic: Make sure all your food is organic. This is the best way to ensure nothing hinders your weight loss goals. Choose organic which will insure that your fruits and vegetables are free of chemicals. If you eat meat, make sure it is certified organic. If not, meat will be full of growth hormones, antibiotics, and other animal drugs. This will totally clog up your system, put tons of animal hormones and chemicals in your body, causing abnormal storage of fat, weight gain, hormonal and

menstrual problems in women, depression, and many other problems. Eat a large salad if/when eating meat to speed up digestion.

Eat Wild Fish: Make sure your fish is wild and not farm-raised.
Farm-raised fish live in small spaces and they are given tons of
chemicals and drugs to increase their growth. They are often also
injected with chemical food dyes to make them look fresher than
they really are. Farm-raised fish diets lead to weight gain and
other hormonal imbalances.

Take Supplements: These oils as supplements should be taken
daily to speed up weight loss.

- **Vitamin E:** improves liver and gall-bladder function, power-
  fully aids weight loss, creates young good-looking skin, and
  keeps arteries open as well as promotes circulation. There are
  good and not so good brands to buy as some have some kind
  of synthetic in them. To get a top quality all natural form you
  can visit the Web site on the appendix page.
- **Omega 3:** This helps with the burning of fat, decreases appetite, helps the liver and pancreas, increases circulation, increases oxygenation in the body, and helps balance hormone
  levels.
- **Acetyl-L-Carnitine:** This helps you burn unwanted body fat
  and is used for fatty acid oxidation. Fatty acids are one of the
  key energy sources the body uses, and oxidation is the process by which they are broken down to create energy! This
  will start to burn your fat off as fuel and energy.
- **Alpha Lipoic Acid:** ALA mimics insulin which may enhance
  the body's sensitivity to insulin. This helps to improve the
  ability of the body to build lean body mass and reduce fat.
  This can be good if you are trying to gain some healthy muscle mass, It also works with creatine to promote energy and

improve your general metabolism and works best in conjunction. The human body does not produce any surplus of Alpha Lipoic Acid naturally, and it is only in this surplus "free" state that it acts as a potent antioxidant. The body produces ALA in very small quantities, due to this fact, those who want the best possible therapeutic benefits of Alpha Lipoic Acid may wish to consider using a supplement. Works best in conjunction with vitamin C and E. It is also a powerful anti-aging and antioxidant supplement. Anyone with Diabetes should only use this supplement if they have the approval of their doctor.

Shower Filter: Your skin is the largest organ in your body. Your water is loaded with fluoride, chlorine, heavy metals, and other chemicals. Showering causes you to absorb more toxins than drinking eight glasses of the same water. So even if you did not drink your tap water but you showered in it, you would still be exposed to toxins. Hot water showers create steam releasing poisonous gas from the contaminated water, which you inhale, getting into your lungs, skin and so on. The best thing to do is buy a good shower filter causing you to shower in pure clean water. That is what I did as soon as I had this information. Your energy levels will come back much higher, dry skin will disappear, and a sense of wellbeing will result.

Massage: During your first phase of doing cleanses and changing your diet, get regular massages if you can afford them—as often as possible—as they will speed up your weight loss; toxins and lactic acid will get flushed out even quicker. Deep tissue is often the best as it goes deeper on a cellular level but most any massage will be beneficial and can directly influence your ability to control or lose weight. Massage has been shown to improve circulation and the supply of nutrition to the muscles and increases tissue metabolism. Massage maximizes the supply of these nutrients and oxygen though increased blood flow and helps the muscles to grow and burn more calories as a result. Waste products such as lactic and carbonic acid build up in muscles during and after exercise. Increased circulation to these muscles helps to eliminate toxic debris buildup caused by these waste products and in doing so shorten recovery time. Massage is thought to be able to burst the fat capsule in subcutaneous tissue so that the fat exudes and becomes absorbed. In this way, combined with proper nutrition and exercise, massage actually helps in weight loss.

Sunlight: Lack of sun slows down your metabolism and leads to weight gain. It also leads to depression, increase in appetite and overeating. At least 20 minutes a day of sun on your face and body is recommended. Moderate sun exposure with the proper protection depending on your skin type is also known to boost your immune system and ward of other sicknesses and certain types of cancers.

Infrared Sauna: The ancients of Finland invented the sauna for healing and cures in ancient times. As I mentioned, the skin is the largest organ in the body. Sweating in a sauna will release fat cells and increase metabolism while releasing toxins, reducing appetite, helping with arthritis and muscle pain, decreasing depression and totally relaxing your mind and body. You can lose more calories sitting in the infrared sauna than even jogging or running for the same length of time but you need to do both for different reasons. You can burn up to 600 calories in just 30 minutes. Detoxification in an infrared sauna is three times higher than in conventional saunas. Sauna use helps to break up cellulite that contains fat! These are the more stubborn fat cells that can melt away in this type of sauna as they go much deeper into the body's layers. Infrared saunas also deeply cleanse the skin often healing up acne, they boost the immune system and a host of other things. I always look forward to my sauna time while unwinding with a good book.

Applying as many of these items to your lifestyle will only increase your weight loss results. The first thing to do is to get on the cleanses and start to eat organic, drink fresh water, and get some exercise. Now you are on your way to super natural health!

ULTIMATE WEIGHT LOSS—HCG

HCG, according to many weight loss experts, is the most effective way to lose weight and keep it off if done in combination with a strict diet protocol. After you have done many of the cleanses and lifestyle changes in this chapter and throughout the book, HCG could very well be the next step in removing the hardest to lose fat deposits, resetting your metabolism, especially for those of you who are overweight and need a powerful jump start in weight loss. It is so amazing that in just three short weeks, it is supposed to reset your metabolism into a fat-burning machine!

What is HCG?

HCG (Human Chorionic Gonadotropin) is a hormone naturally occurring in the urine of pregnant women. However, most HCG on the market today, such as Pregnyl, is synthetic. Christmas Jones explains how HCG works. "In layman's terms, HCG is said to perform a metabolic recovery, where the hypothyroid is said to be reset, boosting the metabolism, and increasing the person's ability to burn fat at a much higher rate. HCG is also said to break down body fat, causing rapid weight loss by mass even before registering on a scale. Simultaneously, it is said to protect the endogenous fat and muscle which the body needs to stay healthy, but also avoiding sagging and loose skin known with excessive weight loss."

In 1954, with the publication of Dr. A.T.W. Simeons' study in the British medical journal, *The Lancet*, HCG was introduced widely to the world as a weight management drug. Dr. Simeons' study and subsequent publication, <u>*Pounds and Inches: A New Approach to Obesity,*</u> discovered that "a small quantity (125 to 250 I.U.) of HCG administered once daily for a short period of time (23 to 46 days) in combination with a very low calorie diet (VLCD) consisting of 500 calories, produced an average weight loss of 1 pound per day." Also, Simeons' work with HCG began the dialogue around the issue of obesity. It was used for the rich and famous in his day.

Today the use of HCG along with the diet protocol is being rediscovered by thousands of people and has found a new resurgence. Every day I meet people who are talking about it and, by doing it, look so much younger and thinner. Many of my close friends who were overweight and have done every diet known to man have found dramatic weight loss, losing more weight and keeping it off more than anything they have ever tried. It is truly amazing to see such effects on the human body. An anti-aging doctor who administers the treatment and prescription told me that it also helps to re-balance and reset your hormone levels. I personally have tried HCG to test it out, more for the natural hormone balancing effects than the weight loss. The result is that, even though I looked very fit, healthy, and exercised regularly beforehand, I lost about 21 lbs. of fat around my waistline and face and kept all my muscle mass. I looked at least 10 to 15 years younger, and my energy was incredible as I was not only feeling lighter but all my hormones were re-balanced, and my metabolism and hypothalamus was basically reset and revved up like I was in my high school days. I was very impressed, and it has basically reversed my age and time clock by about 15 years.

The most compelling components to HCG with the diet protocol according to the experts in this field are:

1. Loss of problem fat (around the abdomen, thighs), not muscle

2. Ability to reset a person's base metabolism so they can process food more efficiently

3. Maintain weight loss

Three Kinds of Fat (from the Pounds and Inches manuscript by Dr. Simeon)

"In the human body we can distinguish three kinds of fat. The first is the structural fat which fills the gaps between various organs, a sort of packing material. Structural fat also performs such important functions as bedding the kidneys in soft elastic tissue, protecting the coronary arteries and keeping the skin smooth and taut.

The second type of fat is a normal reserve of fuel upon which the body can freely draw when the nutritional income from the intestinal tract is insufficient to meet the demand.

But there is a third type of fat which is entirely abnormal. It is the accumulation of such fat, and of such fat only, from which the overweight patient suffers. This abnormal fat is also a potential reserve of fuel, but unlike the normal reserves it is not available to the body in a nutritional emergency. It is, so to speak, locked away in a fixed deposit and is not kept in a current account, as are the normal reserves.

When an obese patient tries to reduce by starving himself, he will first lose his normal fat reserves. When these are exhausted he begins to burn up structural fat, and only as a last resort will the body yield its abnormal reserves, though by that time the patient usually feels so weak and hungry that the diet is abandoned. It is just for this reason that obese patients complain that when they diet they lose the wrong fat. They feel famished and tired and their face becomes drawn and haggard, but their belly, hips, thighs and upper arms show little improvement. The fat they have come to detest stays on and the fat they need to cover their bones gets less and less. Their skin wrinkles and they look old and miserable. And that is one of the most frustrating and depressing experiences a human being can have."

HCG with the special diet is the hottest topic when it comes to weight loss today. The basic protocol is a 500-calorie diet along with HCG taken sublingually or with injections.

However, HCG is not without its detractors and its controversy. The FDA only approves the use of HCG for the treatment of certain problems of the male reproductive system and in stimulating ovulation in women who have had difficulty becoming pregnant. The FDA is adamant that "no evidence has been presented, however, to substantiate claims for HCG as a weight-loss aid." Moreover, the FDA requires all labeling and advertising of HCG used in a weight management program to include the following notice shown here:

"These weight reduction treatments include the use of HCG, a drug which has not been approved by the food and drug administration as safe and effective in the treatment of obesity or weight control. There is no substantial evidence that HCG increases weight loss beyond that resulting from caloric restriction, that it causes more attractive or "normal" distribution of fat, or that it decreases the hunger and discomfort associated with calorie-restrictive diets."

To have the desired effects, it is clearly stated in Dr. Simmons' writings and by the health experts and administering doctors that one you must follow the Simeons protocol exactly as instructed by substituting and eating certain foods as well as refraining from certain foods while on the protocol.

Before starting an HCG-based program and diet, it is highly recommended you do so under the direct supervision of a physician experienced at providing this type of diet to their patients. Also make sure you are taking enzymes and B12 during the protocol. Some physicians do not understand the Simeons HCG weight loss protocol, so you certainly don't want them as your guide. Also remember HCG in its most potent form is normally only available by prescription from a physician. *It's best not to buy HCG from the Internet* or from someone who says you do not need a prescription. Often you have no idea where that HCG is coming from. There seems to be a lot of HCG (and other prescription drugs) coming from questionable facilities in other nations. Any HCG you receive should be from a Federally licensed compounding pharmacy located in the United States or Canada. The little money you will save is probably not worth the potential health risks (or reduction in HCG potency) by buying it from an Internet site (or a weaker homeopathic version that doesn't even need a prescription). Though I do know people that went the Internet route and still lost weight, they claim to have had a much harder time than those with a prescription who breezed through it all. There seems to be an option to order homeopathic HCG or sublingual HCG and then mix it yourself with B12 then refrigerate after opening for those who absolutely cannot find a doctor to prescribe it to them. But I would really take all precautions before ordering anything online as, again, it's best to have someone tracking your progress with the best and most potent form of HCG and have the proper blood tests first to make sure you are eligible for the treatment.

Conditions: According to doctors who prescribe it, men and women at least age 14 and over can take <u>HCG Sublingual Drops, except for those with the conditions listed here.</u>
<u>The following exceptions are:</u>

- **Heart disease**. They need to be stable and have clear ECG for 3 months prior to treatment and periodically during treatment. Obtain approval of cardiologist.
- **Pregnancy/Nursing Mothers**
- **Cancer and/or Tumors**
- **Large uterine fibroids**

As with any diet plan, check with your physician.

Chapter 4

Mind and Thoughts

"Nothing can stop the man with the right mental attitude from achieving his
goal; nothing on earth can help the man with the wrong mental attitude."
—Thomas Jefferson

"As a man thinks, so is he."
—King Solomon,

Just as you are what you eat, you also are what you think. The way
you see yourself is who you become. Every action is based first on
a thought. Once your thoughts start to change—about yourself
and life—your life starts to change. Because actions are the results
of thoughts, to see change you need to allow your thoughts to
be conditioned in a way that will bring you maximum results in
every area of your life. You need to take control of your thoughts
and not allow just any thoughts to dominate your life. Just as
raw food has an energy force, thoughts are so powerful that they
release energy—good or bad—depending on the thoughts.

When you get a strange dream of someone chasing you trying
to hurt you, your heart beats faster and you wake up feeling
exhausted, as if it really happened. Your mind treated it as fact.
When you watch an intense action-filled movie, your mind sends

the same signals to your body as if you were in the car on the high-speed chase causing reactions in your stress levels, heart beat and so on. Your body does not differentiate between whether what you are seeing is reality or simply a movie or dream. As you see the images in your mind or on a screen, your body reacts to them positively or negatively.

Thoughts are creative in nature and if thoughts are consistent enough, they start to manifest into reality. The more you think and focus on a particular thing, the more it will become a reality.

When you start to think about something negative, like how you will pay your bills, or if you will get evicted from your home, or lose your job, your body suddenly starts to release toxins into your bloodstream affecting your heart rate, arteries, energy, immune system, and many other things.

Thoughts of anger, rejection, fear, or bitterness all produce negative effects on your body and your own peace and joy—releasing dangerous toxins into your body. Just thinking about certain negative things can adversely affect your life. Negative thoughts start to spiral you downward—where so much energy is devoted to these thoughts that you are then too worn out and depleted to think and act on thoughts that build you up and drive you to achievement and super natural health. When you often think negative thoughts, people can pick up on that and sense something negative that drains people around you; they tend to distance themselves.

When you live in a constant state of fear and anxiety, this depletes the immune system. Such people will get sick much faster than those who don't live and think this way. Start to think on things that are helpful, exciting, positive, and energizing!

VISUALIZATION

When you see yourself as achieving great health and joy, thinking the best of people and having other positive thoughts, this releases a rejuvenation of your cells; your health improves. If you start to see yourself in great internal and external shape, your mind will send a signal to your body helping you to achieve this or any other goal.

Just as there are laws of gravity and laws of flying (airplanes), there are also laws that affect the natural and spiritual realms. "As a man thinks so is he" (Proverbs 23:7) was written by the great man of wisdom, King Solomon. Thinking you are more than able to attain super natural health or weight loss will cause you to achieve it. If you think there is no way, then that is what you will get. Most sickness can be a result of wrong thinking leading to wrong actions about food choices or emotional patterns that lead to sickness.

You need to take full control of what you allow to enter your mind. If it is a negative thought, quickly replace it with a positive thought of someone that told you they loved you, or when your baby was born, or anything positive that happened in your life. You have to take negative thoughts captive and then send them on their way.

Everything you see around you was first created in someone's mind then came into manifested reality. You are what you think about and how you see yourself.

OVERCOMING PAST THOUGHTS

How do you get rid of negative thoughts that have been there since youth? Many people have been conditioned as kids in negative thoughts from parents, teachers, and other authority figures in their lives—even other classmates.

Maybe a father told you that you would never succeed or did not show the love you needed at the time. You might have been picked on in school. Because this might have been etched into your mind at a very young age, it affected all your decisions or indecisions—affecting your relationships and life. Oftentimes later in life, we discover we have hidden anger or resentment against those blamed for our present lives.

To start changing, you have to first take charge of your life and not let someone else dictate who you were really created to be. The most powerful force in the world is to forgive the person that hurt you in the past so that you can go on and create a new future. Continuing to hold on to what someone said or did, as bad as it was at the time will only limit you and continue to be self-destructive. If you hold onto it, then they win and you become what people told you that you were, but if you let go and forgive, you win and prove to be totally opposite of what was spoken over you as a curse. Once you forgive them it will feel like a million pounds of weight lifted off of you—freeing you from a prison of defeat into a new life of limitless possibilities. Also the original culprit may even sense a new freedom as they may have a hidden or a subconscious sense of guilt for how they treated you. Try it right now and simply say, *"I forgive so and so from what they did or said to me."* Say it several times to imprint it into your psyche and spirit.

Now you are on your way to supernatural health as this is the most powerful thing you could ever do! You will notice a new joy and people will start to be attracted to you because of this new sense of love and forgiveness that will exude from you.

ASSOCIATIONS

If you hang around people who always put you down and are always cynical, critical, and depressed and they don't want to change, you need to make some new friends who propel you toward who you want to be. Guilty by association is true. You take on the positive or negative attributes of those you spend time with. When you hang around with angry people, you tend to be angrier than before, as anger will slowly but surely creep upon you as you tolerate it. *"Make no friendship with a man given to anger, and with a wrathful man do not associate, lest you learn his ways and get yourself into a snare."* (Proverbs 22:24)

FOCUS

Focus on things that are noble and positive.

"Whatsoever things are true, whatsoever things are honest, whatsoever things are just, whatsoever things are pure, whatsoever things are lovely, whatsoever things are of good report; if there be any virtue, and if there be any praise, think on these things." (Phil 4:8)

You always move toward what you focus on. Focus on how you will feel when you achieve this or that dream or goal. Once you start to imagine how you feel, you actually start to tap into the future living the feelings of joy and satisfaction of a future event before it happens. Your mind and body can't always tell if what you are thinking is in the present or future but simply starts to cause your body, spirit, and everything else to react now according to what you are thinking whether it be present, future, or past.

As you strongly focus more on what you are aiming for, your brain will start to work overtime to find the solution in your subconscious while you sleep. Also help from above from the Creator will start to flow as you are in tune with the patterns and laws that govern how things operate in the invisible world. Your mind is like a computer chip that only has so much memory or capacity. If your mind is overly focused on a negative problem—constantly worried about what may happen—your thoughts may be overloaded with fear; even if the solution were to be downloaded to you, there would not be any more room in the memory bank of your mind to receive the message. If the message box on your answering machine is full, you cannot receive the very important life-changing message you are waiting for.

Clear your mind of fear and worry so that you can make room for the solutions that will come to you once you create the proper environment to receive them. Your mind is like a memory card and only has so much memory on it. If it is full of stress, negative things, or it's just full, it's much harder to receive a fresh download from above.

DESIRE

What you think about, often leads to stronger desires. When you couple consistent thinking and desire, they start to manifest into reality. The stronger your desire, the faster you will act on it. Again it all starts with thoughts. If you casually desire to be in good health but are not motivated enough to act on it, then your desire needs to be increased to spur you to action—just like when you might have strongly desired chocolate chip cookies because of a commercial you keep seeing over and over. The result is the same. You run to the store and buy them. If you start to think thoughts of what you want to achieve or see yourself 30 pounds lighter, eventually you will act in accordance with those thoughts. Again, as I mentioned earlier, thoughts and visuals have an effect on the body, mind and spirit. When you dream, while sleeping your body and mind do not always know the difference if what it is experiencing is a present reality or a future tense scenario that you may be catching a glimpse of. The same thing works when watching TV or a movie. Your heart can still race in an intense scene even though it's not occurring in actuality. Even a mental picture that you imagine in your brain can start working for you or against you. See your future and destiny and think of these things even now and on a consistent basis and you will start to attract the necessities, connections, and resources to fulfill it.

SPEECH

What you speak has an amazing effect on everything you do and on your body. Speech is so powerful that it is recorded that everything was created by it. In the beginning Creator spoke, *"Let there be light, and there was light."*

Speech and sounds that you speak, though invisible to the naked eye, are real objects. If an opera singer can sing at a high pitch and break glass, then it is a tiny object—like a pebble—but smaller. At high speeds or frequencies, it can pierce through another object.

Scientists call these "sound waves."

Sound waves created by speech are so small that if you were to divide the smallest particles and atoms up into some of their smallest forms inside these atoms, at its core you would find a vibrating sounds wave called quarks. These sound waves are embedded in everything on the earth including rocks, food, trees, and everything ever created. This means that speech was one of the first ingredients that created everything you see and the invisible things you don't see. This also means that these sounds waves can be altered and respond to other sound waves or speech.

$$E = mc^2$$

Einstein's theory of relativity explains it well as he was way ahead of his time. His theory in simplified terms is E is energy and M is matter or substance. Basically, Einstein was concluding that energy is real and is considered matter even though it is invisible to the naked eye. You cannot see electricity itself but you know it is real when you turn on a light and see its effect. Thoughts and speech release energy. So when you think and speak certain things, you are actually releasing matter or creating things—good or bad.

SOUND WAVES CONTINUED

Studies have been made on water particles and the water particles under certain studies responded to how the scientists spoke to these water particles. In studies conducted by Japanese researcher Masaru Emoto, water particles and other subatomic particles actually respond to sound and even speech or words spoken to it. If this is true, then every created things can hear in a sense and respond in some way as all things created were first created with the same core ingredients—sound and light. In some nations such as Canada, where it is legal, doctors use a procedure called high-intensity focus ultrasound—high-energy sound waves—to destroy cancer cells. These are sound waves, but imagine the power of speech against sickness, especially if you use the highest power source, the Creator's power, when speaking to objects such as disease to vanish.

Start to speak the things you want to see manifest in your life. If you are going for a job, start to say that you are going to have great favor with everyone you meet and you will be success-ful. Start to tell your body that it is strong and healthy and that no sickness can survive in such a healthy state. Sometimes I will even say with great joy and humor that my body is so healthy that sickness does not feel comfortable around me and just has to leave. This actually according to even quantum physics, science, spiritual giants, and the ancients seems to all confirm each other. Start to create your day—each morning—by speaking what you believe will be created, that you will be successful in all that you do, that you are full of energy, and that you will have favor with everyone you meet after connecting first to the Creator's power and love. This will cause things to shift from the invisible realm to the visible realm and will also take you from natural to super natural health. Your health will be determined, in large part, by how well you control and bridle your speech to create health and life. *"Death and life are in the power of the tongue, and they that love it will eat its fruit"* (Proverbs 18:21).

FOOD AFFECTS THOUGHTS

When you eat foods that are not natural and continue this process all the time, the dead foods that you eat that are not energy foods will start to drain you and make you feel less energized. This feeling of being drained will lead to feeling grouchy, negative thoughts, and complaints. So what you eat does affect your thoughts eventually. And your thoughts affect what you eat.

For instance, a lack of an amino acid called tryptophan can lead to depression. Tryptophan is found in raw, high-protein foods such as goji berries, spirulina, chlorella, blue-green algae, maca root, cacao, and other raw foods. Through cooking, tryptophan is destroyed as it is sensitive to heat. Meats contain this amino acid, but if you eat only cooked meat and potatoes (bad combination for digestion), the amino acid is destroyed. Start to incorporate lots of raw foods into your diet and see the difference it makes!

Chapter 5

Stress-Free Living

"Don't worry about anything; instead, pray about everything.
Tell God what you need, and thank Him for all He has done."
(Phil. 4:6)

Most people today admit to being stressed. People are stressed mentally, physically, and emotionally. Stress has been proven to weaken your immune system, increase weight gain, and cause many sicknesses if not managed and drained out.

Stress is not an illusion or figment of your imagination or simply an emotion; it can actually be measured, when under stress your body reacts and changes. Some of the changes are a rise in blood pressure, faster heartbeat, adrenalin production, faster breathing, and increased blood and sugar pumped to your fingers and toes.

When someone feels threatened they go into a fight or flight mode, usually flight mode—a desire to run away from the threat of real or perceived danger. Stress can be good and was ingrained into the human system by the Creator—made for real life-and-death situations like escaping from a lion or bear in the jungle or forest. Sometimes to meet an urgent deadline, the stress factor will kick in and you begin to operate at peak performance as an athlete or on the job for a certain goal or accomplishment, which you can then easily recover from.

Stress was never meant to be an ongoing daily way of life. This is where it gets dangerous. Ongoing stress is harmful as it releases toxins otherwise known as "stress toxins" clogging up your entire system if not drained out. Exercise is the fastest way to release stress but if you are being chased by a lion as our ancestors might have been before the modern age, then those toxins would have already been released from the exercise of vigorously running away. When you have this type of stress on an ongoing basis and don't release it with exercise or deep relaxation, then your body is clogged up with toxins making your immune system very weak and wide open to stress-related diseases—high blood pressure, cancer, ulcers, heart attacks, diabetes, and much more.

Stress affects not only the body but the mind. Your mind can only handle so much in its memory banks. When you are stressed by a perceived problem like your boss calling you into his office or someone not returning your phone call for an important meeting that could get you fired when in fact they simply lost their cell phone or the boss called you in just wanting to congratulate you or it might have only been to ask a simple question. The perceived threat and the fear of not knowing and thinking the worst possible outcome can create stress for many people.

When you are stressed, your mind is so obsessed and focused on the fear of what could be that you start to block everything else out. You start to neglect your body and get into bad habits of eating and sleeping. Stress can affect your relationships making you irritable and paranoid—thinking that everyone is out to get you—over-reacting to everyone else. This adds conflict that only multiplies the stress you already had with more emotional stress— taking you down a slippery road. You need to take control of it.

Stress really in its simplest form is living in FEAR. Most of the time when you feared the worst and stressed, things were almost never as bad as you thought they were, they were worse—no just kidding, they turned out to be nothing most of the time.

Perception makes the difference. One person's positive perception is another person's worst nightmare. The one with the positive outlook stays happier and healthier living a longer more productive life.

THE PERFECT STORM

Often times a combination of small stresses can lead to an overwhelming sense of hopeless stress. Things like your car breaking down, then getting laid off, family member sickness and finding out your retirement account just lost half its value—all at the same time—can cause The Perfect Storm. **Our perceptions cause our stress.** It's our perception of the event, and not the event itself that causes our stress. What causes you stress may not even faze me—and vice versa.

What are the most important ways to manage stress?

1. **Exercise vigorously**. It's important to get the kind of regular, vigorous exercise that your physician approves of.

   Every once in a while, you'll hear someone say that we have such a high rate of stress-related illness in our society today because we have so much more stress to deal with, but there are researchers who believe that we aren't dealing with any more stress than our ancestors did. They believe that the high rates of stress-related illness happen because our lifestyle doesn't include the vigorous exercise that earlier generations automatically had. Exercise basically cancels out the effects of the stress reaction on our bodies by draining off the "stress toxins."

2. **Relax regularly.** Another effective stress management technique is to use deep relaxation, which neutralizes the negative effects of stress. Practice the relaxation response for about

20 minutes a day in a comfortable position. Praying and singing to the Creator also really works. A good massage and being outdoors in the sun similar to a day at the beach relaxes you and gives you a different outlook.

3. **Realize that your attitudes and perceptions play a key role in managing stress**. Most of the things you fear the most never happened. Change your perception and think the best, don't always expect the worse because what you believe as fact often comes to you as you can create it even by your thoughts. Believe in the best and realize that you are probably overreacting.

4. **Have realistic expectations.** Many of us create our own stress by setting our expectations unrealistically high. This is especially true if you are a perfectionist. Plan out bite-sized things that you know you can do and then check them off once finished, giving you a sense of accomplishment. Do what you can and write out your plan for the following day the night before. Then, once something has been accomplished, check if off as "Done."

5. **Arrange your life so you feel in control.** You don't have to be in control, you just need to feel you are in control of your schedule and your lifestyle.

   Plan how you will start to solve the situation and then do at least one of those things right away. If the creditors are harassing you daily to pay an outstanding bill then take control, don't let them control you. Call them up and tell them what you can pay within the next week or two and start from there. Then you will start to have a sense of control instead of letting others and stress dictate how your day will go.

6. **Build and maintain a working support network.** This is the system that supports you in times of need and makes you

aware that you're part of a bigger whole toward which you, too, have a responsibility.

Support networks are particularly important when you're under stress. Remember that one of the problems caused by stress is tunnel vision—an inability to look at alternatives and options. Stress also makes you feel paranoid—people are trying to get you or that they're purposely being difficult just to aggravate you. Share your perceptions with the important people in your life to see if you're seeing things clearly. Ask them if they see the situation the same way you do. Do they have ideas about what you can do about it?

7. **Spend time with your loved ones.** We know that strong families tend to spend time together often. Unfortunately, when families get under stress, a natural tendency is for the individuals to go off on their own or to lash out against those closest to them. Don't shoot down your only allies!

One of the healthiest things a family can do when under stress is to purposely plan to spend some time together, to go for a walk, or just get out of the house and do something fun together outdoors.

8. **Balance your commitment to your children—your job— your loved ones—yourself.** Either too much or too little emphasis on ourselves is unhealthy, but we can constantly search for that happy middle ground for both ourselves and our families.

9. **Only you can determine the amount of stress that's good for you.** The amount of stress you need to operate effectively, at your very best, is very personal. Figure out what is the best amount of stress for you and then monitor it so that you don't take on less or more than is healthy and productive for you.

ELECTROMAGNETIC STRESS

Staying indoors too much actually can cause bodily stress. Especially when you are in a place that has many electromagnetic waves—those from cell phone, computers, appliances, ovens, airports with heavy electromagnetic interference from the control towers and so on.

Stress from these waves is caused by electromagnetic radiation called EMF (electromagnetic frequencies) caused by magnetic fields. Appliances and cooking have EMF but they dissipate the further you are from the source—the kitchen. But high-powered sources of EMF, such as powerful transmission towers and lines, travel up to hundreds of feet right through walls. The same applies when you are around many devices that are plugged into your wall.

EMF is invisible—yet so damaging and harmful—and has been shown to cause cancer. There is a great deal of evidence out there proving this. According to the *New England Journal of Medicine* in a report from 1982, utility workers were reported to have double the incidence of leukemia compared to men in other occupations. Other reports show a major connection with EMFs and the incidence of leukemia, lymphoma, and cancer of the nervous system in children. The EPA has tried to warn the public, but the powers that be realize the huge financial loss in utility and other industries if the entire infrastructure of the modern world had to be changed.

What do you do? There are still ways of protecting yourself. Try not to sleep right next to electrical gadgets especially those with higher EMFs that plug into a wall outlet. Keep appliances a good distance away from you—on the other side of the room or in another room—cell phones, computers and so on.

CELL PHONE DANGERS

These are the ones to watch out for the most. Cell phones emit levels of radio frequency (RF) in the same range as microwaves causing electromagnetic radiation. The cell phone industry even admits that cell phones are not safe as Motorola said, "It is well known that high levels of RF can produce biological damage through heating affects…" The same User's Guide of the Motorola company says, "A few animal studies, however, have suggested that low levels of RF could accelerate the development of cancer in laboratory animals. In one study, mice genetically altered to be predisposed to developing one type of cancer developed twice as many such cancers when they were exposed to RF energy compared to controls."

The User's Guide goes on to explain similar studies on humans! It goes on to say about humans being affected, "**When tumors did exist in certain locations, however, they were more likely to be on the side of the head where the mobile phone was used.**" It continues, "an association was found between mobile phone use and one rare type of glioma, neuroepithellomatous tumors."

I have noticed, when holding a cell phone for too long on one side of my head, at times a sharp pain can result, draining me of my energy.

Cell phones are known to interfere with pacemakers. Even the Nokia 6560 User's Guide states under Additional Safety Information: "Pacemaker manufacturers recommend that a minimum separation of 6 inches be maintained between a wireless phone and a pacemaker to avoid potential interference with the pacemaker." It advises people with pacemakers not to carry the phone in their breast pocket and to hold the phone opposite the pacemaker.

If this can occur with pacemakers, I don't want to be a statistic years down the road as people realize cancers and other diseases are caused by improper use of cell phones. These phones also drain your energy. Cell phones are manageable for short calls but were not designed for longer use. Here are several recommendations to limit your exposure to cell phones. First, throw your phone away, just kidding again. . .

1. Always put the speakerphone on and stand a few feet away and use a home phone for longer phone calls.

2. Buy a radiation-free headset. This is the only headset I know of that has no radiation. Normal headsets send the radiation right to your ear. The radiation emitted from your wireless radon-free tube headset keeps the radiation away from your brain. Even cordless home phones are dangerous as they send the radiation to the cordless phone device. Put the speaker-phone on, and keep the phone at least a few feet away when talking instead of putting the phone up to your ear.

3. Buy a Bio-pro Cell Chip for your cell phone and computer—devices most people use regularly. These are little chips that you stick to your phone; they are known to neutralize the dangers of radiation from electromagnetic frequencies (EMF). I always have one on my phone.

4. Buy a Q-Link necklace. These devices worn as a pendant reduce the harmful effects of electromagnetic frequencies generated from cell phones, computers, and other devices. As I travel a lot by plane near people with all kinds of wireless devices, air traffic control towers and so on, I have noticed that the Q-Link gives me a major increase in energy and I bounce back quickly after my many speaking trips. It takes a day or two to get used to; I have so much more energy. World-class athletes have noticed improved mental focus and endurance giving them a competitive edge when wearing the Q-Link.

5. See a chiropractor. Often the stress of a back that is not aligned can add more stress in your life and also affect your nervous and immune system. In the past 3 decades, the field of neuroimmunology has published a significant amount of

research showing a connection between the nervous system, the immune system, and subluxations of the spine. It removes lactic acid and removes stress as will a good massage.

6. Walk Barefoot. There is a new stress-free trend, and it is walking barefoot! Not only will it help you relieve stress, it has been noticed that people who have walked barefoot in their childhood encounter fewer foot troubles as compared with those whose feet were always covered with slippers, sandals, or shoes. In other words, the children who go barefoot and are allowed to do so by their parents have been seen to have fewer foot deformities, greater flexor strength, and more feet agility. At the same time, they are able to spread their toes to a greater extent than others.

Irrespective of the extent of care the shoe companies take in making footwear that suits the shape of human feet, they can never ever beat the comfort that one gets from barefoot walking. In fact, those who walk with their shoes on encounter much more aches and pains in the body as compared with the people who indulge in home barefoot walking.

Benefits of Walking Barefoot

1. Barefoot walking helps straighten out the toes of a person. At the same time, if you walk barefoot, even the lazy muscles of your feet are prompted to move and develop more, with the result that you have toned and much stronger foot muscles.

2. Another positive effect of barefoot walking that most of people are unaware of is that it helps the leg muscles pump blood back to the heart. This makes it beneficial for those who are suffering from the problem of varicose veins.

3. Though most of the people are unaware of the fact, walking barefoot helps relax tired feet. **It has also proven beneficial**

for people suffering from flat feet, in many cases helping them overcome the problem altogether as it works the muscles that are never used in the foot and some have claimed to have had arches formed from walking barefoot. Shoes often protect the feet so much that certain foot muscles get lazy because they're not being used. The best Olympic runners are from Kenya, and they all train barefoot.

4. Walking barefoot in the summer season has been found to have a cooling effect on the body of a person, especially if he/she walks on morning grass, leaves, or a piece of log in the garden.

5. In traditional exercises like the martial arts, it is believed that being barefoot helps a person stay more connected and focused. Also when you walk on the earth barefoot, you connect with the Earth's natural vibrations which helps to ground you in some way as those walking on the beach. As you walk with your feet bare, you increase your vitality. At the same time, it helps you think clearly and increases your capacity to work.

Walking barefoot in your garden or the local park will help you feel closer to nature and cause stress to diminish like a day at the beach. This will not only take your mind off everyday tensions and relax your body, but also rejuvenate your mind and boost your energy levels. There are now special minimal shoes that have been made to help you start walking barefoot. Even flat-footed people have claimed to be cured in time!

Whatever you do, start slow as your feet will get sore quickly at first as the muscles are not used to being worked. Usually you walk with your heel first with normal shoes but walking or running barefoot causes you to typically land on the ball of your foot towards the lateral side. Start by walking around the house barefoot or in your yard. Then slowly try walking for maybe half a mile and gradually build up to longer lengths until you can do more. It should cause an overall healing effect; connect you more with the energy of the Earth; diminish stress on your feet, legs, and body; and cause an overall feeling of relaxation and freedom as you go throw off your restraining shoes!

THE REST PRINCIPLE

Even the Creator rested on the 7th day. If you work non-stop seven days a week, you will burn out. You need to take a day to completely cut off from work, cell phones, computers, and anything that causes stress. It is often referred to as Shabbat or a once a week sabbatical. Spend that day resting, rejuvenating by talking to the Creator, spend time outdoors, read, and meditate with music. That day of rest will cause your other six days to be twice as productive. This is how humans were made; those who rest at least once a week have better physical, mental, and emotional health when they take a day to be with themselves, family, nature, and the Creator. You deserve it!

Chapter 6

Foods That Heal

*"Ninety per cent of the diseases known to man
are caused by cheap foodstuffs. You are what you eat."*
—Anonymous

Raw foods can be an amazing medicine for the body and allow for mind-boggling levels of energy, health and vitality.

Once, my immune system was severely attacked. I was not sleeping enough and over-exerting myself in work and exercise for a few weeks. I suddenly became very weak, had a severe sore throat with bumps on my head and near my ears; my lymph nodes were swollen. I was sweating a lot. Basically, my immune system was in need of a major reboot and I needed lots of rest. What I needed in this case was to fast and only drink in miracle foods for maximum healing. When you refrain from eating, your body focuses all its energy on healing instead of on digesting. That is why you want to liquefy these foods in a blender or juicer. Here are some miracle foods that helped me to quickly cleanse and heal. They acted as a natural antibiotic when I was in need.

RAPID IMMUNE SYSTEM BLEND

1 ripe orange habanera pepper (or a ripe jalapeno): You will feel this cleans you with a fire-like sensation through your body as it kills bacteria and viruses. It also will start to clear out your nasal passages of mucus almost immediately.

2 cloves of garlic & 1 slice of ginger: Garlic and ginger are natural antibiotics that boost the immune system when weak. Ginger also helps reduce swelling in the throat. These two are power twins for infections.

6 figs: Figs are amazing at dissolving mucus and cleansing the gastrointestinal tract helping to detox your body.

1 handful of parsley or kale: Both of these are rich in iron, which builds strong red-blood corpuscles.

2 organic apples (or 4 organic pears):   Apples and pears contain pectin that helps to remove toxins; they help with bowel movements, which drains the lymphatic system and alleviates the swelling in a sore throat and tonsils.

1-ounce organic cold-pressed, extra virgin olive oil: Olive oil helps to build strong white blood corpuscles.

Because I am a motivational speaker addressing crowds across America and around the world, on the rare occasion when my throat is sore, it is imperative that I get healed ASAP the healthy way. I make myself a powerful miracle tea that alleviates the pain. I will even stop over at a health food store and go to the deli to get the warm water, then add these ingredients. This is what I do at the first sign of any of these symptoms.

Colloidal Silver. Another way to boost your immune system is to take certain powerful natural supplements. Colloidal silver is a dietary supplement made of pure silver and distilled water, and which, throughout the centuries, fulfilled multiple functions.

Hundreds of years ago, the pharmaceutical market was basically at its beginnings and, instead of antibiotics which is prevalent today, people used natural products to prevent infections. Apparently, colloidal silver was one of the top products, due to its efficiency in supporting the immune system. With the expansion of the medical world and consequently, the pharmaceutical industry, colloidal silver's use did not increase. On the contrary, laboratories and specialists have discovered new uses of the product, such as stress relief, skin conditioner or better physical performance.

The rich concentration of silver molecules in colloidal silver basically destroys bacteria and viruses and keeps the immune system safe and sound. Moreover, products based on colloidal silver are non-toxic, nor do they lose power to act when in contact with other antibiotics or medical treatment. The silver component has been proven to be compatible with the human body and no tolerance limit has been found to prevent people from using it.

Furthermore, the use of colloidal silver does not have to be long term, as in the case of antibiotics medication. Colloidal silver does not impose any long-term treatment. This happens because of the fact that silver particles destroy viruses and germs from the first contact and, this way, bacteria and other human body microorganisms do not have time to develop a firewall against colloidal silver. As strange outbreaks of viruses are occurring this is one of the best ways to stay healthy and protected.

Echinacea and Goldenseal are another dynamic duo of the herb kingdom that I take when travelling or feel something coming on! The extract is helpful for naturally boosting and fortifying the defense ("immune") system, purifying the blood and lymph fluids, strengthening and toning all the major organs and glands, and helps to repair damage to the major eliminative channels by cleansing the tissues,

Astragalus

Complex polysaccharides present in astragalus appear to act as an immunomodulator. Immunomodulators possess the natural ability to increase the body's production of messenger cells that regulate the immune system. The overall effect is a more efficient immune system. Studies on astragalus indicate that it can prevent white blood cell numbers from falling in people given chemotherapy and radiotherapy and can elevate antibody levels in healthy people.

Reishi Mushroom

Though used in Traditional Chinese Medicine for at least 2,000 years, only recently has reishi mushroom received much attention due to its apparent immune-enhancing activities. Studies have shown that reishi may transform many components of the immune system including NK cells. Moreover, one study concluded that reishi's effect on such immune-related cells as T and B cells yielded further evidence that **reishi's value comes from it's ability to enhance immunity response**.

Immunity Formula: A new supplement called *Immunity Formula* combines all of these super immunity supplements in one by *SuperHealth* vitamins. It actually contains all the immunity ingredients you would need including echinacea, reishi mushrooms, garlic, zinc, korean ginseng, magnesium, selenium, riboflavin and vitamins A,C, and E.

Healing a Sore Throat

6-to-8 ounces of warm water (preferably fresh spring water)
Squeeze ½ lemon

*Fresh raw ginger, a few pieces cut up or 1 tablespoon of ginger
  powder*
Raw Honey—1 teaspoon or tablespoon

Flus and colds are common. Most people will run to the pharmacy but I have noticed that as you cleanse your body, it does not respond well to the pharmaceutical medicine that ends up clogging your system. Raw natural foods act as a potent source of healing without the side effects. Below is what I do at the very first signs of an oncoming flu or cold. Try drinking this blend on an empty stomach three times a day, replacing meals for a few days or at least for a 24 hours period and see how fast you heal. It's pretty amazing to say the least.

Natural Flu and Cold Medicine

4 oranges: Peel oranges but keep the white pith. Oranges and papayas are an excellent antioxidant.

1 papaya: Skin the fruit and remove all seeds. Both of these fruits will cleanse out the toxicity, which is what leads to a weakened immune system. They also help cleanse your intestinal tract and are full of calcium and rich in vitamin A, beta-carotene, and vitamin C.

6 Figs: Take off the stem and make sure they are soft. These are one of the best mucus dissolvers.

Optional

1 hot pepper, jalapeño, or orange habanera pepper: Cleanses out sinus cavities and bacteria. Hot peppers contain phyto-antibiotics that wipe out bacteria-causing sickness.

1 avocado: For added thickness to offset the hot peppers

For those who would love a meal replacement that is full of energy, strength, and stamina and that tastes good, here is what I do almost daily!

Super-Food Energy Blend ('Maca Chaca' *Drink*)

Wild Young Coco Water: You can either buy a fresh coconut and pour the water and the flesh or even buy canned coconut water at the health food store with the flesh to save time, though wild is always better. Coconut water hydrates your body more than even water and cools down the body especially in hot or tropical locations.

Gogi Berries: (1 small handful) These are the highest antioxidant energy foods on the planet because they grow in the highest altitudes on the earth—places like Tibet—and are able to withstand the harshest climates where almost nothing else grows. They contain at least 18 amino acids and are a complex protein as well as an excellent source of minerals—they taste great!

Raw Chocolate Powder: (1 tablespoon) This type of chocolate actually is full of many raw nutrients and helps with weight loss as it inhibits appetite and tastes awesome! You can also replace raw chocolate powder with raw chocolate nibs.

Maca: (1 teaspoon or tablespoon) This food helps to regulate hormones, increase energy, and increase testosterone in men and progesterone in women. Maca is rich in minerals and increases vigor and affects your mood positively.

Spirulina: (1 teaspoon or tablespoon) This has one of the highest concentration of natural protein (along with chlorella) on the earth! This algae was consumed for thousands of years by the original peoples of Mexico and Africa.

Benefits of Goji Berries

- 500 times more vitamin C by weight than oranges
- Has vitamin E, which is nearly unheard of in fruits
- More beta-carotene than carrots
- Contains B vitamins
- Helps increase testosterone and libido
- Has 19 amino acids which include 8 essential amino acids
- Has 21 trace minerals, which include zinc, calcium and selenium
- Contains beta-sitosterol which aids in lowering cholesterol and improves sexual health
- Has anti-bacterial and anti-fungal properties
- Has essential fatty acids such as Omega-6
- Has anti-cancer properties

SPIRULINA

Spirulina is a single celled blue green algae, that contains 10 vitamins, 8 minerals, and 18 amino acids. (essential and non-essential). It contains a complete protein of 65–71%, that is 12–15 times more protein than steak and is 5 times easier to digest than meat or soy protein. It has been found to help reduce weight, and help with many allergies, visual problems, carbohydrate disorders, anemia and many other disease conditions. It also has many beneficial enzymes. This "super" algae is a deep blue-green color because of the chlorophyll and phycocyanin. The green pigment is caused by chlorophyll, which is sometimes called "green blood" because it is so similar to hemoglobin.

Spirulina Facts

Several years ago, the National Cancer Institute announced sulfolipids from blue-green algae like spirulina were remarkably active in test tube experiments against the AIDS virus. In 1993–95, research showed natural polysaccharides in spirulina increased T-cell counts, strengthened the immune system and raised disease resistance in chickens, fish and mice. The animal feed industry is embracing spirulina as a new probiotic to replace overused antibiotic drugs in animal feeds. In 1994, a Russian patent was awarded for spirulina as a medicine for reducing allergic reactions from radiation in the Children of Chernobyl, the rare essential fatty acid GLA, sulfolipids, glycolipids and polysaccharides.

Its deep green color comes from its rainbow of natural pigments—chlorophyll (green), nutrients are absorbed quickly.

Spirulina Is The World's Highest Beta Carotene Food, Reducing Long-Term Health Risks

Spirulina beta carotene is ten times more concentrated than carrots. So even if you don't eat the recommended 4 to 9 servings of fruits and vegetables every day (most people eat only 1–2), get your natural beta carotene insurance from spirulina to help support your body's defenses.

Spirulina Has A Rare Essential Fatty Acid That Is A Key To Health

Gamma-linolenic acid (GLA) in mother's milk helps develop healthy babies. Studies show nutritional deficiencies can block GLA production in your body, so a good dietary source of GLA can be important. Spirulina is the only other whole food with GLA.

I always mix spirulina into my raw food smoothies. It is also great for those who want to cut down on meats or for vegetarians and raw foodists as it's the most potent plant protein.

Spirulina contains Cobalanin or B12 (2mg/kg) B12 is one of the most difficult of all vitamins to obtain from a plant source. Spirulina contains 250% more B12 than beef or liver.

Spirulina also contains 8 essential amino acids: Isoleucine (4.13%), Leucine (5.80%), Lysine (4.00%), Methionine (2.17%), Phenylalanine (3.95%), Threonine (4.17%), Tryptophane (1.13%), Valine (6.00%), 10 Non-essential amino acids, Alanine (5.82%), Arginine (5.98%), Aspartic Acid (6.34%), Cystine (0.67%), Glutamic Acid (8.94%), Histidine (1.08%), Proline (2.97%), Serine (4.00%), Tyrosine (4.60%), 8 Minerals, Potassium (15,400 mg/kg), Calcium (1,315 mg/kg), Zinc (39 mg/kg), Magnesium (1,915 mg/kg), Selemium (0.40 ppm), Iron (580 mg/kg), Phosphorus (8,942 mg/kg), Pyridoxine or B6 (mg/kg), Biotin (0.4 mg/kg), Pantonthenice Acid 11 mg/kg), Folic Acid (0.5 mg/kg), Intositol (350 mg/kg), Niacin (118 mg/kg), Riboflacvin or B2 (40 mg/kg), Thiamine or B1 (55 mg/kg), Tocopherol or v E (190 mg/kg), (Carotenoids which produces Vitamin A), Alpha-carotene Beta-carotene Xanthophylis Cryptoxanthin Echinenone Zeaxanthin Lutein.

Chlorella

Chlorella has been touted as the perfect whole food. Aside from being a complete protein and containing all the B vitamins, vitamin C, vitamin E, and the major minerals (with zinc and iron in amounts large enough to be considered supplementary), it has been found to improve the immune system, improve digestion, detoxify the body of toxins, mercury and heavy metals, accelerate healing, protect against radiation, aid in the prevention of degenerative diseases, help in treatment of Candida, relieve arthritis pain and, because of its nutritional content, aid in the success of numerous weight loss programs.

Chlorella contains ten to 100 times more chlorophyll than leafy green vegetables. It is grown in a controlled medium where minerals are added to optimize it for human consumption. Its small size requires centrifuge harvesting and special processing to improve the digestibility of the tough outer wall, which makes it more expensive than spirulina. However, chlorella's cell wall binds to heavy metals, pesticides, and carcinogens such as PCBs and escorts the toxins out of the body, making it a particularly valuable supplement. Use as directed.

I find chlorella especially helpful during a cleanse and especially useful during colonics as it attaches to the cell walls of your intestines pulling out impacted fecal matter and hard to remove toxins. Chlorella is probably one of the best natural defenses against cancer. I take it daily in tablet form especially when I travel. There are several papers on the prevention and/or inhibition of cancer using chlorella as well as documentation of its DNA repair mechanism.

ORGANIC PURE GRASS JUICE

Organic pure grass juices like wheatgrass, barley grass and alfalfa deliver high concentrations of valuable nutrients including vitamins, minerals, naturally occurring enzymes, and chlorophyll. Moreover, this alkalinizing effect will promote healthy pH balance in the body. Typical diets that include processed foods like white flour and sugar, coffee, and soft drinks cause a pH imbalance in the body and become too acidic. Too much acid in one's body will decrease the body's ability to absorb nutrients and minerals, decrease the energy production in cells, and make the body more susceptible to illness and fatigue. Therefore, maintaining a healthy pH balance is necessary for optimal health and wellness. Wheat grass alone is so powerful not to mention the other grasses but let's look at a few benefits of wheat grass.

Blood Benefits

Wheatgrass and organic pure grass juice tablets may help clean the blood of impurities. It is said to increase the red blood cell

count and lower blood pressure. Wheatgrass may also en   .ge
the body's metabolism and enzymes to work more efficiently and
increase blood flow.

Stomach Disorders

Wheatgrass tablets have been used to treat diarrhea, constipation, colitis and certain ulcers. It is also suggested for stomach
pain and distress.

Turn Back the Clock

Wheatgrass tablets **may help restore gray hair to its natural
color**. It is also used as a kind of youth tonic to help keep the
body young, alert, energized and fit. Some say it enhances fertil-
ity in both men and women.

Anti-Inflammatory

Wheatgrass tablets contain the enzyme SOD, which claims to reduce the harsh side effects of radiation. This enzyme is also useful
in protecting cell damage, especially after a heart attack.

Fight Tumors and Toxins

Wheatgrass tablets may be able to ward of toxins and even fight
tumors. The compounds found in wheatgrass help cleanse the
blood and counteract toxins that may invade the body. Because
I travel often and don't always have the time to make it nor do
I always like the taste of liquid grass juices like wheat grass but
love the incredible results they bring to my immune system I take
them in organic tablet form from *SuperHealth*. Their 100% organic and vegan *Pure Grass Juice* tablets that I personally take
contains a proprietary "superfood" blend of the best of the best
grass juices like alfalfa, barley, kamut, oat, and wheat grass juices
to deliver all the best potent concentrations of key vitamins, minerals, and nutrients.

You can order one of the best organic spirulina, chlorella and organic grass juice supplements from *SuperHealth* at **super healthvitamins.com.**

Healing Power of Coconuts

Coconuts are one of the most amazing superfoods on the planet. I drink coconut water daily as the water base to all my shakes and raw drinks as it's the most complete hydrating liquid a human can consume. Here is why:

The water and flesh from young coconuts contains the full range of B vitamins, with the exception of B6 and B12. B vitamins are essential for providing us energy as they break down carbohydrates and proteins. They also support nervous system function and, interestingly, the muscle tone of the stomach. Young coconut water is also high in minerals, particularly calcium (for bones), magnesium (for the heart), and potassium (for muscles).

- Coconut water is more nutritious than whole milk—less fat and NO cholesterol!

- Coconut water is better than processed baby milk; it contains lauric acid, which is present in human mother's milk.

- Coconut water is naturally sterile—water permeates through the filtering husk!

- Coconut water is a universal donor—it's identical to human blood plasma—**this is the most amazing benefit**! Some nations use this for blood transfusions when they run out of blood donors! In fact, it was regularly used during WW II for wounded soldiers when blood plasma was low.

- Coconut water is a natural isotonic beverage—the same level we have in our blood. I have found that it is more hydrating than water or any electrolyte sports drink.

In fact, this is how many survive on coconuts in hot jungle-like tropical climates. It not only hydrates but also cools down the body temperature while energizing you. My favorite coconut drink, which can be purchased with or without the coconut flesh in the water, can be found in many health food stores like Whole Foods or New Frontiers which you can buy all natural and canned to take with you on trips.

Coconuts also help in weight loss. The effect on your thyroid from coconuts is shocking; they can boost thyroid function by up to 20 percent. Having an efficient thyroid is essential for our bodies to carry out several functions including boosting our metabolism and energy production.

> In the 1940s, farmers tried coconut oil to fatten their animals but discovered that it made them lean and active and increased their appetite. Whoops! Then they tried an antithyroid drug. It made the livestock fat with less food but was found to be a carcinogen (cancer-causing drug). In the late 1940s, it was found that the same antithyroid effect could be achieved by simply feeding animals soybeans and corn.

Coconut also is a potent antibacterial and antifungal agent; it is a great cleanser of our guts and is something that can help heal the gut should problems like leaky gut syndrome occur. On top of this, coconuts will help your body fight off infection so it's a great thing to eat when you are unwell or feel something coming on. It is converted to monolaurin by the body, which fights off infections (viral or bacterial).

Cancer Fighter
It keeps getting better—coconuts have been proven to have anticancer effects especially of the colon and breast. This is due to the oil's protective nature and ability to safeguard the body from infection while cleansing your system.

SUPPLEMENTS THAT HEAL

Supplements that you should definitely include in your arsenal are **Saw Palmetto** for men.

Saw Palmetto is a popular "men's herb," Saw Palmetto is used primarily as a treatment for enlarged prostates. As **many** as 50% of **men** experience symptoms of an **enlarged prostate** by age 60. One man in six will be diagnosed with prostate cancer during his lifetime, but only one man in 30 will die of this disease.

Prostate cancer is the second leading cause of cancer death in men in the U.S. Time and money invested now, will pay huge dividends later.

COQ10

It is not only found in every cell in the body, it is **needed by every cell in the body.** Here is a list of its key benefits:

- Helps treat congestive heart failure.
- Helps improve nerve function.
- **Fundamental to energy production at the cellular level with mitochondrial strengthening.** (The mitochondria is the part of the cell responsible for creating energy.)
- CQ10 is an important element for the creating cellular energy.
- Gives protection against strokes.
- Improves blood pressure.
- Improves skin by slowing down the skin's aging process; this is due to its potent antioxidant. capability in destroying free radicals. It is an **anti-aging** compound.
- One study suggests it may help improve glucose control in Type 2 diabetics.
- Another study said that a 400 mg dosage helped to incur cancer remissions, including prostate and breast cancer.

TRANSFORMING YOUR BODY

The human body is the most amazing creation. Our bodies are always trying to re-create. Our bodies re-create themselves every day. Many in the field have stated that 98 percent of the atoms in our bodies are replaced every two years. Studies have shown that 100 percent of our atomic structure is replaced every 7 years.

When you change your eating and living habits by eating organic, raw, green alkalizing, and highly mineralized foods, you can speed up this process altering your bones, skin, hair, weight, and internal organs, re-creating and re-building your atomic structure into what the Creator intended humans to look and feel like.

Of course in this process you will also be re-building and helping to release and activate the most important aspect of your being which is your spiritual as well as mental, emotional, and physical state, which are all inner-connected.

Chapter 7

Beautifying Foods

"Don't be afraid to be amazing."
—Andy Offutt Irwin

Secret foods that emperors, kings, actors, and models have used for a long time still exist today. They are beautifying foods. You can eat these directly or juice them.

CUCUMBERS

The Roman Emperor Tiberius was known to love cucumbers so much that he ate 10 of them every day. Though native to western Asia, they were very popular with the Egyptians, Greeks, Romans, Sumerians, and Romans. Alexander The Great introduced them into Europe; Christopher Columbus introduced them to the Americas.

Cucumbers are one of the most beautifying foods—especially if you blend them with celery and apples as a juice drink. Cucumbers are an excellent source of silica, which is a trace mineral that contributes to the strength of our connective tissues.

Connective tissue is what holds our body together. Cucumbers are effective when used for various skin problems, including swelling under the eyes and sunburn. They also contain ascorbic and caffeic acids. These acids prevent water retention. That may explain why when cucumbers are applied topically they are often helpful for swollen eyes, burns, and dermatitis. Cucumbers have a high water content and low sugar which is perfect as a beautifying food inside and out, especially for skin. Because they also have natural saltiness, it helps to transport their juice into the tissues, hydrating the body at a deeper level. They also are a great kidney cleanser. Their enzymes—erepsin—help to digest foods and proteins and aid in killing tapeworms. The silicon and chlorophyll in the cucumber skin greatly improves skin complexion. (Must be organic if eating the skin.) Cucumbers are a perfect food as they are hydrating, low calorie, alkaline, high energy, cleansing, and skin beautifying.

PAPAYAS

Papayas are very beautifying as they enhance skin beauty, nail strength, and hair luster. They contain large quantities of calcium and vitamin A as well as high levels of collagen-healing vitamin C. Besides eating them to help against Acne you can also apply a mask using the fleshy side of a green papaya skin on the acne. Papayas are also one of the very best foods for digestion. They have been found to reduce heart attacks and the risk of certain strokes such as arteriosclerosis partially due to the capaine, an alkaloid compound. They also contain antitumor and anticancer properties. Half-ripe papayas are often prescribed for raw-food eaters due to the low sugar content which is recommended for cancer. Also, their higher enzyme content helps with weight loss and flatulence. When I am in Hawaii surfing my absolute favorite food is Hawaiian papayas for breakfast before I go ride some waves.

MSM (METHYL SULFONYL METHANE)

MSM is made of sulphur. It benefits skin hair and nails and has a beautifying effect on them as it smoothes the skin because of its collagen building effects, strengthens hair and nails and causes acceleration of hair growth, promoting lustre. It is an essential component of all connective tissue. It is the vital component in the formation of keratin, collagen and elastin, giving flexibility, tone and strength to our muscles, bones, joints, internal membranes, skin, hair and nails. Sulphur can clear acne sometimes in a matter of weeks. Its effects are accelerated by adding Vitamin C such as Camu Camu powder or capsules.

It is also a free radical scavenger. MSM can give a relief of swelling, inflammation and pain and symptoms of arthritis and research has shown that sufferers improved their symptoms. This is a pure and beneficial form of organic sulphur, a naturally occurring nutrient found in every living organism.

In its purest form, it is white crystals and is a naturally occurring mineral. MSM is a beneficial dietary supplement of sulphur. It's toxicity rating is the same as water, and it has the lowest levels of toxicity in biology. It can safely be taken in accordance with the instructions on the bottle with other medications, although it is always recommended that a doctor be consulted before you take *anything* in addition to your prescription medication. It is best to start with the lowest dose and build up. The lowest recommended beneficial amount of 1500 mg per day, in 2 or three doses, although some people are taking as much as 10,000 mg quite safely in the specific treatment of arthritis although it also benefits skin, hair and nails. When I'm busy and travelling I use MSM in capsule form. I also like to buy it in it's purest form as white powder then mix vitamin C as the two work great together and it tastes much better that away. It can take from a couple weeks to a few months to start seeing the effects a your body needs time to get used to it. If you do it first thing in the morning its easier to get into a habit of taking it.

CELERY

Celery is especially great for your skin as it can clean the skin cells, dirt, and remove skin oils. It not only can help you to fight against acne, but also dilute the acne scars. It is extremely efficient to people who want to loose weight and maintain their health. The exceptional benefits of celery have been recognized for centuries by ancient medical practitioners. Even Hippocrates, the father of medicine has claimed that celery has a major role in calming the nerves. Celery neutralizes the organism, promotes the proper functioning of the immune system, it purifies our body and keeps it in a balance. Furthermore, it is a great source of calcium, which helps to build strong teeth and bones and celery also provides your body vitamin A. Celery is a great source of B vitamins such as B1, B2 or B6, giving you energy for a fresh start of the day. It is also high in nutrients such as magnesium, iron, folic acid and potassium contains plenty of water, therefore it provides a proper hydration for blood cells. Due to its high water and potassium content, celery is used for cosmetic purposes being a highly effective plant for treating dry, dehydrated skin. Celery rehydrates the body and helps to maintain a healthy libido.

AVOCADOS

Avocados are amazingly healthy, despite their bad rap for having too much fat. Yes, they do contain up to 15 percent of the daily-recommended amount of fat, but it's the good fat—the polyunsaturated and monounsaturated fat that actually helps to moisturize our skin and keep us feeling satisfied. You put it on your face in mask form which does wonders for your skin, so why not try actually eating it and see the benefits. Eaten in moderation the monounsaturated fats you ingest will give clear, soft and smooth skin.

They contain folate, which helps blood formation and is essential for cell regeneration and the oil that avocado extracts aids in triggering the production of collagens. So incorporating more avocados into your diet will mean less wrinkles and a more tone, even skin appearance. Avocados are rich in potassium (60 percent more than bananas), vitamin A, Vitamin E—an effective fat-soluble antioxidant vital to the normalcy of our body's functions, and B vitamins, which help with metabolism and energy levels. Look for the bright green skin. The brighter the fruit the more beta-carotene they contain, so look for vibrant green ones that are slightly soft to the touch. If only harder, unripe avocados are on offer, just allow them to ripen in a brown bag for two to three days.

WATERMELON

Watermelon's rosy complexion is courtesy of lycopene (also found in tomatoes), which has been linked with a decreased risk of some cancers and is a skin soothing antioxidant that protects the skin from oxygen damage. Oxygen damage can weaken the skin's outer layer and that makes it easier for acne causing bacteria to thrive. As if that wasn't enough reason whet your appetite for watermelon, it also has some other pretty amazing beauty benefits. Its luscious fruity aroma is not the only reason it has become a ubiquitous ingredient in many natural beauty products like lip balm, shampoo and exfoliators. Watermelon juice protects skin from the suns harmful rays and the acids in those juices can act as a natural exfoliant on skin, which also help to clear it free from blemishes, and can aid in the regenerative process of skin cells.

ONIONS

They may not be the most romantic food out there when it comes to your breath, but after hearing the benefits that onions have on your skin, a few missed kisses will be worth the sacrifice. Besides adding flavor to food, their therapeutic properties and benefits might interest you more than their taste. Onions have antibacterial and antifungal properties that will ultimately bring beauty to your skin. They are full of sulfur—they actually contain more than one hundred sulfur-containing compounds (these compounds are why we tear up when cutting onions), which helps cleanse the skin by purifying the liver. A cleaner liver will ease food digestion and keep blood flowing properly throughout the body. Since one cup of onions provide you with 20% of the recommended daily intake of chromium, a bacteria-reducing mineral, onions will aid in the battle against acne, too.

Silicon

Silicon is a mineral with remarkable healing, regenerative and beautifying properties. It is highly concentrated in hair and nails, and is also present in skin, teeth, connective tissue, muscles, bones, cartilage and lungs.

Silicon has the incredible ability to transform into calcium. Therefore, a silicon-rich diet leads to an increase in bone mineral density, beautiful teeth and jaw formation, and helps to reduce tooth and gum decay.

Studies have shown that the oral and external application of silicon improves the condition of aging skin, hair, and nails in women. Silicon increases the thickness and strength of the skin, improves wrinkles, and gives hair and nails a healthier appearance.

Silicon plays an important part in the formation of connective tissue. Consequently, it helps to maintain the elastic quality of the skin, tendons and generally, of cell walls.

You can increase your intake of silicon, by consuming the following silicon-rich foods: cucumbers (with skin), bell pepper (with skin), tomatoes (with skin), radish, romaine lettuce, marjoram and nopal cactus.

Zinc

Zinc is necessary for the proper function of several enzymatic functions important for healthy skin. Zinc is essential for a beautiful skin complexion since it is necessary for the functioning of enzymes that digest damaged collagen and rebuild new collagen.

Zinc promotes cell division, repair and growth. It helps the lymphatic system to oxygenate the tissues and eliminate wastes properly. It also works synergistically with other minerals and vitamins. For instance, Zinc in combination with sulphur and vitamin A, helps to build strong hair.

You can naturally increase the levels of zinc in your body with consuming the following zinc-rich foods (preferably raw): pumpkin seeds, pecans, cashews, sunflower seeds, sesame seeds, coconuts and pine nuts. I like to take natural zinc supplements to make sure I have the right amount in my system besides eating the raw organic foods that contain it.

BEAUTIFYING SUPPLEMENTS
DMAE

DMAE's most promising benefits is that it **promotes healthy skin**, by stopping the process of arachidonic acid being manufactured, which is a substance that can lead to wrinkles and aging of the skin. Some of the functions of DMAE also include the **improvement of concentration and memory**. It reduces the appearance of wrinkles, age spots, and other problems that come with age. It may also treat autism, memory deficits, depression, and dementia. It may treat sleep problems, Alzheimer's, and ADHD. Some sources of DMAE are oily fish such as sardines. DMAE can lift ones mood level to a more positive side, counter depression and bad moods, and raise and improve cognitive functions (such as memory and concentration), DMAE can even increase intelligence. Small amounts are produced in the body. However for many people, supplementation may be necessary. It is best to check with your doctor if you think you need to take DMAE but you can buy it without a prescription. Physician's closely watching patients on DMAE have reported that such people are more upbeat, and have greater positive mental acuity. Also, people taking it often, have reported sleeping deeper and having much more energy when awake.

Vitamins C and E

These power twin supplements can give your face a lift without a face-lift! How? In a nutshell, they significantly improve skin's health because they counter the damaging effects of sun exposure. We are all exposed to the sun whether we're sun worshippers or not—simply leaving the house without sunscreen can cause skin to age prematurely and become dry and wrinkled. Even worse, prolonged sun exposure can lead to skin cancer. Your skin needs vitamins C and E desperately, every day. So what should you do? To give your skin a robust vitamin C treatment from the inside out, eat foods that are extra rich in vitamin C, such as citrus fruits (oranges, grapefruits, lemons), bell peppers (green and red), broccoli, cauliflower, and dark leafy greens such as spinach, kale, and mustard greens. You might also beautify your skin by taking vitamin C supplements, between 500 and 1,000 mg per day.

Vitamin A

This vitamin is also an essential vitamin to include in a skin-care regimen. If you don't have enough vitamin A, your skin looks dry and flaky rather than young and healthy. Vitamin A maintains and repairs skin tissue; so adding it directly to your skin can result in a real improvement. You may notice your acne disappearing, your wrinkles smoothing, and your psoriasis lessening, all because of a skin-care cream rich in vitamin A. An acne-free, wrinkle-free, rash-free face is truly beautiful.

Vitamin B

Vitamin B complex may be the most important vitamin for your skin. Biotin, found in B vitamins, is a nutrient that forms the basis of skin, nail, and hair cells. Without enough biotin, your skin will lack radiance. Be sure to get your biotin by eating foods such as oatmeal and bananas and apply biotin directly on your skin in a cream or lotion. The result: Your skin will transform, shimmering with a healthy glow, as it retains moisture, stays smooth, and looks younger—all in less than a week!

Vitamin K

This supplement is also a big blessing. Nothing looks less healthy than dark, puffy, under-eye circles. To eliminate dark circles under your eyes and reveal beautiful, glowing skin, try using a vitamin K cream or supplement.

This combination of beautifying superfoods and natural vitamins can reduce photodamage from the sun's rays, smooth wrinkles, keep skin moist, and enrich its texture, making it—and you—healthy and glowing.

Hair, Skin & Nails: This supplement actually contains many of the key beauty ingredients mentioned above all in one supplement which is great for those with a busy life. It contains things like silica, collagen, vitamin, A, C, E and many other key ingredients for maximum beautifying effect which is available at *superhealth vitamins.com*

Chapter 8

Creating Your Future

"If you can imagine it, you can achieve it;
if you can dream it, you can become it."
—William Arthur Ward

The invisible world is more real than we think. In fact, it is what determines what occurs in our visible world. Recent studies in quantum physics have discovered that subatomic particles will begin to change form simply by being observed by humans. As in the case with water particles, when they were spoken to in a certain way, they would change form according to either angry words, love or other words connected with a certain emotion.

Everything created on this earth is made up of core subatomic particles that can be altered by human observation—amazing! Just thinking about certain things immediately causes either a positive or negative effect on your body, whether its angry thoughts releasing poisons or happy loving thoughts releasing healing.

If this is true then objects in the invisible world change and re-create by simply being observed or even thought about. By observing something that is in your future and looking and thinking about it, invisible subatomic particles will start to shift causing things to come your way from potential to reality. Whatever you think about and speak starts to be created.

When you get a creative idea or inspiration and start to think about it more intensely, something is already being created. Then when you start to speak and declare that you will do this or that, the reality of it starts to speed up even faster toward fulfillment and soon after action follows on your behalf. Before you know it, you run into someone or get a phone call that is the open door into the very thing that started as a download into your brain—a creative thought from the Creator. You become what you think and speak about.

It is even recorded in the book of Genesis that the Creator spoke and then things were created. This makes more sense today given the scientific language and discoveries to explain how this could be possible.

YOUR BRAIN IS A RADIO TRANSMITTER

Many do not realize that the human brain acts as like a radio transmitter sending out frequencies. Have you ever thought about someone you needed to call for a few days and suddenly they called you as they said they were thinking of you for the past three days? When the intensity of thought is strong enough it sends a signal to other brains. Everything is made of atoms, protons, electrons and frequencies including thought and speech.

If sounds like an opera singer can sing and release invisible sounds waves at a certain pitch and break glass so can a strong enough thought start to create sub atomic particles in the form of frequencies.

An experiment was made to prove this point. Every object has a certain amount of frequency coming out of it. In one experiment they took a bar of gold and aimed radio frequencies at the gold bar. When they measured the frequency on the gold bar, they discovered that the vibration and frequency of the gold changed when a radio wave or x-ray was aimed at it. Next they experimented with a person intensely aiming his thoughts also on a gold bar. What they discovered was after the thoughts were aimed at the gold bar the vibration and frequency emitting from the gold bar was equally changed due to the strong thought frequency aimed at it sent from the brain.

Thoughts can send out a weak signal or a stronger signal. Have you ever suddenly been hit with a very heavy dark sad feeling wondering why as there was no natural situation that would have caused you to feel that way. Then shortly afterwards you discovered someone was very upset with you and was not only intensely thinking thoughts about you but speaking negatively about you. Now you discovered why? Also the reverse occurs when you feel this sense of excitement like something really good is about to happen but you don't know why or what. A few days later you realize that a decision had been made on your behalf that was very favorable for you. You already received the frequency being transmitted days before the actual reality hit you.

Our brains transmit energy on different frequencies. You can transmit with as much power as you choose. When your brain transmits frequencies through your thoughts it is picked up by other brains that have the ability to pick up such signals. What you think about also affects physical matter. I heard a story of a doctor that mixed up the results of two different patients. One patient had full blown cancer and had three months to live. The other patient's tests showed he was cancer free. The doctor accidently switched the results. When the man that was cancer free was told he had three months to live immediately his brain began to send very strong signals that indeed there was a cancer. He thought about it day and night, his emotions believed it and his actions confirmed it as he planned his funeral. Within three months he actuality developed terminal cancer and died. The other man that actually had the cancer mistakenly was told that he did not have cancer. His brain began to send signals of healing. He started to dream again of all the things in life he wanted to accomplish. He cancelled his funeral plans and began to be thankful that he was healed and was a better person for it thanking the Creator he was given a second chance. When he was checked again three months later the cancer had gone into remission and he was cancer free. Both these patient's brains released very powerful intense radio type frequencies which in turn created responses and signals in the body.

Just thinking about something that makes you angry, sad or negative can get your immune system to start shutting down, your heart starts to beat faster, your blood rushes to your face and negative toxins are released into your bloodstream clogging you up just from toxic thoughts of anger, resentment, bitterness, rejection and the like. It's not that you will never experience these thoughts but it is how fast you dispose of them. One rule of thumb is never go to bed in this state of mind, release it before you sleep so that it does not get into your system all through the night. The best way is to simply say out loud "I release this situation and I release and forgive that person." Next discipline your mouth not to speak about it because if you continue speaking about it your words will re-create the situation and the thoughts start to kick in again re-creating the past all over again along with the toxic emotions that come with it.

Another interesting concept is that if objects and people can pick up thoughts and words imagine the power of thoughts and words if a person is in meditation or prayer and connected to the Creator. Then imagine the power of those words compared to someone not connected to a higher power. It seems throughout history the words of certain people's words carried much greater power than the average person to where people are spellbound when they speak. Some of the most famous people in history had such power when they spoke as it was backed up by very intense thought frequencies backed up by yet a powerful spiritual force they received in personal times of reflection or meditation despite hard times. These are the words and phrases that today are used in everyday language once coined by such people that knew the power of thoughts and words. Thoughts and words if used correctly can create situations that did not otherwise exist.

WORDS THAT CREATE

Once your goals and destiny are observed and thought about consistently, the invisible framework starts to create circumstances for it to become reality. Now its time to kick it into turbo mode! Words that are spoken with absolute belief, faith, and certainty will start to bring unity of focus and create those very words. If for example, you casually say, "I will become an A-list actor" but your thoughts and beliefs are not congruent with what you just said or believe, this causes imbalance and hinders it's visible manifestation. Others might say, "I will lose 30 pounds by this date and be in the best shape possible and nothing will stop me!" If you speak with total conviction, passion, and clearly visualize yourself thinner and healthier, then you are going to see it happen. You have incorporated all of yourself—words, thoughts, passion, and emotions at a higher level, together in unison.

When you speak something intending for it to become reality, what percentage of power are in those words? Is your mind, body, passion, and focus 100 percent when you are speaking? Or are you speaking something with maybe only 10 percent belief, thoughts, and intensity of belief. To the degree that your mind, emotions, thoughts, will, passion, and words are all congruent with high intensity all at the same high level will determine the speed and probability of that which you are speaking to occur.

Basically if you can unite your mind, body, will, emotions, and actions all on a high level of energy and focus, there is not much that can stop the thing you are aiming for into become reality.

PASSION

When you are totally passionate about something that you feel or know you are supposed to do or become, things start to come your way. The level of emotion and intensity or drive is a huge determining factor in seeing it to reality. You have to want something bad enough to do something about it.

Action on your part to cooperate with your vision or destiny usually does not come without an intense internal force called passion. For some people it's getting a report from a doctor that they have cancer or some other sickness that serves as a driving force to change their lifestyle. To others it's not so much a negative that drives them, but a glimpse into the future of the joy they will feel when they are lighter, thinner, and more energetic. That joy of who they can become starts to increase their passion and drive!

You can go through all the steps mechanically and still miss the mark if there is not a sense of excitement, drive, and passion in whatever you undertake to accomplish. If you could do anything in life and money was not an object, what would you do? Start to work toward that thing in life that naturally drives you and you will accomplish so much more than trying to do things that others expect of you, which do not necessarily motivate you. This is a huge secret to success—in finding your purpose in life, helping to add passion to passion.

Everything produces itself after its own kind. Apple seeds produce apples; orange seeds produce oranges; and on and on since the beginning of time. You have natural talents and abilities that you were born with. Start to use those gifts and talents to help others and you will have a great sense of fulfillment. This will also draw you closer to the Creator. So many people just exist and do not passionately live life to the fullest. They have not tapped into what they are destined to do or realized their natural talents, gifts, and desires; the world is waiting for their release.

BLOCKAGES

Often times we associate a certain goal with pain and suffering. Maybe the last time you went on a diet or tried to exercise, something went wrong and you ended up gaining more weight or hurting yourself in a gym. Then a book like this comes along to really help you but there are these mental and emotional memories of past experiences that block you from taking action. It's like your conscious mind is saying yes—wow this is great! But then by the time you are about to take action, all these fears and blocks hinder your progress associating this with past failure.

You have to re-program your mind and body. You can do this by starting to associate change with pleasure, imagining how good you will feel and look, not by what happened last time you tried something new. Also program your mind by reminding yourself of all the sicknesses you will avoid by starting on this new supernatural health lifestyle. The same is true for anything in life if you can associate it in a positive light to motivate into action.

When a woman is pregnant or has had lots of pain or complications at childbirth she may start to say and think that "this is the last time I am going to do this". But then as time goes on as she is enjoying her new baby, she starts to dream again of the joy and pleasure a second child would bring to her, her husband, and her first child. The pain associated with childbirth gets replaced by many more positive memories of the new baby as time goes on. This leads to having the faith to overcome the negative programming and lots of positive associations with a second child.

Other cases can be when someone applies for a new job or an aspiring actor auditions for a new movie or TV show. Sometimes the fear or perception of a past rejection hinders some from moving on and accomplishing great things. Those who can remove the negative past associations will be driven to action by the joy set before them of the accomplishment and joy that will be derived once they are hired.

Start to work from the future to the present. Imagine you already have that job, career, book published, healthy leaner body and so on. How do you feel now—as if you have already arrived at your greatest dream right now? As you start to see, imagine, feel, and enjoy right now what the future will be feeling it now, you are actually accelerating its existence—already tapping into the senses you would feel as if it already occurred! You don't have to wait until the future becomes a reality to actually enjoy the senses and joy of what that will be like. Your body and mind, as I mentioned before, do not know the difference between a future mental image or something occurring now. As you start to see your future and even feel the joy of that goal, you will be tapping into your future now! Then all the other details will start to fall into place. You will get more insight on the next step to take and before you know it, you will become that which you already started to think about and enjoy.

The secret is to first **define your dream** or goal and then have **100% passion** and get your desire and excitement at full throttle about that dream. Then have **100% belief** that what you are seeing will and is happening and being created then take **100% action** towards that goal knowing that it is happening and is out there waiting for you to simply act on it and realize it! Action is where many people stop. You can dream about it and talk about it but until you finally take action it will be an unrealized dream.

Start taking a baby step right now toward that dream, it may be a phone call, writing the first page of your book or auditioning for a movie or even starting a business by creating your new business idea's legal structure and name on legalzoom.com as if you already have a business. The rest will fall into place. As you take your first step the next step will be clearer as things and the right people and connections will start attracting themselves your way. Take your future now and bring it into the present by enjoying, celebrating, and seeing yourself already there!

Chapter 9

Age Reversal

"...who satisfies your mouth with good things,
so that your youth is renewed like the eagles."
—King David

One of the least talked about subjects is the brain and how it affects everything in your body. The brain is the control center of everything. Once you learn how to feed and utilize this control center, you can literally start to see drastic changes beyond any diet and begin to experience age reversal!

Once you are able to get a handle on brain food you can greatly control your weight and an entire host of other conditions avoiding things like dementia and Alzheimer's disease, reversing the aging process.

The body is actually designed to re-create itself. Every year your body re-creates itself. In fact 98 percent of the atoms in your body re-create themselves every year. Every month your skin is totally renewed. Every three months your skeleton is re-created. Every 5 days you have a new stomach lining. Even brain cells that cause you to think helped create carbon, nitrogen, and hydrogen and those same substances were not there 1 year ago including the raw material that creates your DNA (deoxyribonucleic acid) that is renewed every 6 weeks. DNA is the fundamental building block for an individual's entire genetic makeup.

Aging starts to occur in the brain. As you age certain chemicals in your body start to diminish. As these diminish, they send a death code to other parts of the body. If you can revitalize these brain chemicals to the same levels as when you were younger, you can slow down and even reverse the aging process. For example, when a woman's ovaries start to die, they send a death code to the rest of the body to start aging at an accelerated pace. When you address the ovaries and bring them back to their normal state, it starts to actually "resurrect" other body parts; life and re-generation come back to its more youthful state. It all starts with brain health.

The idea is to first find out what part of your body is aging the fastest. Once you repair one part of the body through brain health, the other parts start to heal and reverse even before you start working on them.

BRAIN POWER

The brain is the control center and transmits signals to your body. As you age, these signals slow down unless you purposely wake them up. You can break the death code in your body by resurrecting and enhancing certain brain functions. There are four key chemicals the brain uses to control the aging process. They are dopamine, acetylcholine, serotonin, and GABA.

Dopamine

Dopamine controls the voltage and power of your brain and its ability to process information. Voltage determines your metabolism, which determines your weight, ability to process food, and level of consciousness and alertness. Dopamine controls voltage, movement, and emotional response. People with Parkinson's disease for example have very low dopamine levels.

Low dopamine affects every area of your body. Low dopamine is one of the fastest age accelerators, sending a signal to the rest of your body to start slowing down and aging—toward sickness and death.

Cardiovascular: When dopamine is low it causes strain on the heart making it work harder than it is used to. Weight gain and fatigue also set in as this lack of dopamine increases blood pressure. If left unchecked, low dopamine could start to lead to a clogging of your vascular system clogging up blood vessels and even leading to stroke.

Immune System: Low dopamine begins to affect your immune system. You start to gain weight when dopamine is low. When you have excess fat due to low dopamine it hinders your body's ability to fight off viruses and bacteria that lead to sickness. Obesity speeds up every type of cancer in every organ of your body. Hormone loss is a major age accelerator.

Menopause/Andropause: Menopause can accelerate to start earlier in women who are heavier or too thin due to lower dopamine levels. Andropause, which is a male form of menopause, occurs in men who are overweight due to low levels of dopamine—leading to low libido and sexual dysfunction and low testosterone. For both men and women it also can also be characterized by depression and low energy. It is like puberty in reverse. If you can control your dopamine levels and keep your weight down, it can take 10-to-15 years off your age. Loss of testosterone results as muscle turns to fat, first in the abdomen area, then the rest of the body.

Things that deplete dopamine levels are stress, poor nutrition, poor sleep, antidepressants, drug use, as well as alcohol, caffeine, and excess sugar. So what do you do to increase your dopamine levels?

Exercise: It increases your dopamine levels immediately. Dopamine increases your desire to exercise increasing the energy in your body. The more you exercise, the more you cause age reversal as your body and hormones start to think it is young again, reversing the death cycle signals. Just 30 minutes of exercise a day will start to reverse the aging process and increase dopamine levels. Exercise will reduce cortisol and stress, strengthening the immune system. It increases circulation to the skin cleansing the pores through perspiration. Exercise also increases muscle-fat ratio, increases bone density reducing risk of injury, and helps sexual dysfunction—increasing blood flow to the organs. As I mentioned before, your body does not know the difference between past, present, and future. The way you see things and act is the way the body responds. Make sure you are doing different types of exercise such as cardiovascular (walking/ running), weights, and so on.

Supplements that will help increase dopamine are: Tyrosine, grape seed or pine bark, gingko biloba along with vitamin C and E and other antioxidants. They help increase dopamine as well as blood flow and energy, focus, and impulse control.

Foods that increase dopamine are almonds, avocados, bananas, raw dairy products, lima beans, pumpkin seeds, and sesame seeds. *Avoid foods* such as sugar, and refined foods along with saturated fats and cholesterol as they interfere with proper brain function and can cause low dopamine levels.

Acetylcholine

Acetylcholine improves memory, concentration, and cognition; it increases blood flow to the brain. It also governs brain speed determining how quickly the electrical signals are processed. When you increase your brain speed by increasing acetylcholine your memory, attention span, IQ, and even behavioral patterns improve. When you are low in acetylcholine, this can lead to dementia, Alzheimer's disease, and learning disorders. Your brain starts to dry up when acetylcholine is lacking; acetylcholine controls and maintains hydration. When you lack acetylcholine your brain speed slows down.

Your brain and body start to dehydrate once you are low in this hormone, which regulates your immune system. Then your bones start to lose calcium as your brain tells your bones and cartilage to provide moisture leading to bone loss, osteoporosis, and arthritis. What is needed to avoid all this is simply to boost your brainpower by keeping your acetylcholine production up, thus reversing this process of degeneration. That is why people with Alzheimer's and osteoporosis are usually frail as the moisture loss in their brain leads to bone, cartilage, and muscle loss to compensate. Lower brain speed leads to cognitive mental disorders. Here are some supplements you should start taking to boost acetylcholine:

Acetyl-L-Carnitine: This boosts acetylcholine, prevents loss of brain cells, slows rate of cognitive deterioration, provides cells with energy and provides cells with brain health. It is also great for converting fat to energy.

Also consider choline, DMAE, fish oils (omega-3), CLA (conjugated linoleic acid), Goto Kola, and gingko biloba, *(As with all supplements, there are precautions that you must be aware of and acknowledge before taking any of the said supplements although supplements like DMAE for example have no known side effects. Gingko is a blood-thinning agent; if you are on any other blood-thinning agents such as aspirin or warfarin, then do not take these before consulting a physician.)*

Also change your diet. If your brain is drying up and you start craving fats there is a good reason—dehydration. Start eating these healthy fats to boost your system with choline. Some of my favorites are avocados, raw goat cheese, cucumber, zucchini, lettuce, poached eggs, and asparagus.

Spices.   You also need spices to boost your brain speed, giving your brain a big boost. Some of these include tumeric, sage, mint, black pepper, basil, lemon rosemary, cayenne, and curry (curcumin), which you can add to your food. India has very low amounts of dementia and Alzheimer's disease, which many believe are the result of the high spice content of their food. Studies have shown that dementia and Alzheimer's caused by amyloid plaques formed in the brain have diminished and/or disappeared when humans have been fed large amounts of the curry spice, curcumin. Mice also had these plaques vanish. Spice intake is encouraged along with regular exercise.

Serotonin

In the central nervous system, serotonin is believed to play an important role in the regulation of body temperature, mood, sleep, vomiting, sexuality, and appetite. Low levels of serotonin have been associated with several disorders, notably clinical depression, migraine, irritable bowel syndrome, tinnitus, fibromyalgia, bipolar disorder, and anxiety disorders. Lack of serotonin makes you feel irritable, depressed, and simply unhappy. Lack of sleep is often associated with low serotonin levels.

One of the fastest way to increase serotonin is to sleep. When you sleep peacefully and long enough you wake up feeling refreshed; a lot of negative emotions often diminish with a good nights sleep. Serotonin levels increase once you are in a deep sleep and help to replenish and renew just about any part of the body. Have you ever felt totally hopeless and frustrated and then took a nap or woke up the next day and the issue that seemed like a mountain did not seem that big of a deal? That's what higher serotonin levels and sleep can do. Also, the creative side of your brain is activated when you rest and sleep more.

When you are overworked and do not sleep enough, this shuts down your creativity, awareness, joy, peace of mind, and affects your personality. Lack of sleep also increases phobias, fear, and nightmares. Lack of sleep is a major age accelerator. Lack of sleep can cause a weakened immune system, bone loss, skin dehydration, poor circulation, decline in memory and mental awareness, depression, and other complications. Also, those who sleep better and know how to rest or meditate can tap into the creativity, new ideas, and even a spiritual state much faster than those who don't. Basically a good night's sleep is like pushing 'reset' on your computer when it's going haywire.

According to Dr. Braverman in his book, *Younger You*. it takes at least about 7 hours a day of good sleep to boost your serotonin levels. Less than 49 hours a week of sleep starts to accelerate the aging process! Some basic things to help you sleep would be to not drink caffeine especially in the evening, avoid electrical things at night such as TV, computers, video games, and the like. Instead read a good book or listen to calming music before sleeping. Avoid naps during the day as this will keep you up later each night.

You can also take natural supplements like melatonin, tryptophan, vitamin B6, fish oils, magnesium, and vitamin B3. (Talk to your health expert or physician about these and any other advanced treatments or supplements.) Some natural foods that help to increase serotonin levels are oatmeal, blueberries, poached eggs, and cottage cheese.

Herbs and spices that boost serotonin are:

Black pepper *(aids in epilepsy, sinusitis, and digestion)*
Cayenne pepper *(helps with neuropathy, pain, headaches, and rheumatoid pain)*

Thyme *(controls spasms, respiratory problems, and fungal infections)*

Turmeric *(protects liver and is a natural body cleanser)*

Basil *(helps lower stress)*

Peppermint *(helps relieve fatigue and tension)*

Borage *(reduces inflammation),*

Nutmeg *(helps with psychotropic properties and alleviates gastro-intestinal problems),*

Sage: *(helps relieve fear, paranoia, and delusions).*

GABA

GABA is a chemical in the brain that causes relaxation, reduces anxiety and stress, and increases alertness; it is sometimes called the "peacemaker" chemical. GABA keeps all the other neurotransmitters and hormones in check.

People who are deficient in GABA can become irritable, unfocused, experience chronic anxiety and have difficulty handling the day-to-day stresses of life. Symptoms of this deficiency can also include headaches, palpitations and heart disorders along with low sex drive, and hypertension.

Though it is true that people often takes prescription medications that can help the GABA receptors, often unfriendly side effects can be the result. The best and safest way to go from natural to super natural health and naturally boost your mood is to go the natural healthy way with diet, natural supplements, and spices.

Dr. Eric Braverman, an expert on brain chemistry and author of *The Edge Effect: Achieve Total Health and Longevity with The Balanced Brain Advantage*, explains, *"GABA is also involved in the production of endorphins, brain chemicals that create a feeling of well-being known as 'runners high.' Endorphins are produced in the brain during physical movement, such as stretching or even sexual intercourse."* As endorphins are released, you begin to feel a sense of calm, often referred to as the Endorphin Effect.

Foods that increase GABA levels are almonds and tree nuts, broccoli, bananas, lentils, brown rice, spinach, oranges and other citrus fruits, halibut, rice bran, whole grains and walnuts—to name a few.

Supplements that also help boost GABA levels are L-theanine; it calms nerves without drowsiness. It also increases mental clarity. This amino acid is also found in green tea, which is an excellent way to start the day off instead of coffee.

GABA has a slightly sedative effect, which is great when taking it before going to bed.

Melatonin is also very helpful in this regard for sleep. All our hormone levels start to decline as early as our 20s including melatonin. With less of it, we don't sleep soundly as we get older with less and less of it in our system. Actress Suzanne Sommers takes a whopping 20 mg per night and claims to sleep better than ever. Contrary to what many think, melatonin has no known toxicity risks, either. You won't overdose on it. The normal cycles of melatonin production are altered due to factors including aging, medications, and light exposure at night. While the long-term health effects of disrupted melatonin secretion are not yet fully known, some scientists have suggested that years of working nights could lead to adverse effects—even cancer.

Fortunately, melatonin supplements can safely and effectively restore balance to the body's circadian rhythm of this important hormone—helping you enjoy a restful night's sleep and keeping your biological clock ticking throughout a long, healthy life span.

Resveratrol—The Anti-Aging Supplement

It has the power to slow down aging, prevent cancer, infections, and even protect your nerves against breaking down.

Needless to say, resveratrol is an excellent supplement against people who are aging and who are suffering from different health disorders that cannot be cured by simply taking those prescription drugs that are very expensive and riddled with side effects. Now onto the anti-aging part—resveratrol's power when it comes to slowing down aging lies at the fact that it can activate a class of longevity genes found in the body that are known as sirtuins. The health benefits and anti-aging potential of reversatrol have been seen and traced NOT only by the medicinal formulations of drugs in Japan and China. According to researchers and doctors, it is the answer to the mystery known as the French Paradox. Despite indulging in foods and dishes that contain 3 times more saturated fat than the usual American diet, the French people enjoy the lowest occurrences and deaths related to cardiovascular problems. And it's all thanks to the red wine (an integral part of the French Diet) that contains high doses of resveratrol. For those of you who are not familiar with it, sirtuins reduces the cellular decay while imparting greater power to your cells for repairing themselves. Matter of fact, many scientists suggest that this type of gene exists in all forms of living organisms and the benefits they bring can be likened to calorie restricted diets—enhance cellular respiration and boost your body's metabolism.

It also slows down the cellular decay, reduces cell death, restricts the multiplication of abnormal cells, gives you more power to repair at the cellular level—all of these and more are important enhancers of longevity and you can find all of these benefits within resveratrol.

Human Growth Hormone (HGH)
What is HGH?
HGH is an endocrine hormone produced by the anterior portion of the pituitary gland. It is made up of 191 amino acids. Production of GH decreases as we age. Virtually every system in

the human body is in some way dependent on HGH for proper functioning. Growth hormone peaks during adolescence and decreases dramatically thereafter. At age 40, our GH production is only 40 percent of what it was at age 20.

It has been shown that as we age, our bodies' natural GH (growth hormone) production decreases. Many of the effects of aging are seen as a result of this decrease. More important, clinical evidence and recent medical research clearly demonstrate that by replacing Human Growth Hormone (HGH) in deficient adults, we can significantly eliminate these symptoms, reverse the biological effects of aging, reduce body fat, increase lean muscle mass, strengthen the heart, and improve sexual performance. No other substance known to medical science has been shown continually to deter and reverse the process of aging.

HGH is produced at a rate that peaks during adolescence, at a time when normal growth is accelerated. The production of HGH decreases with age, 14 percent each year, on average. Humans normally produce about 500 micrograms of HGH daily at age 20. By age 80, the daily production falls to 60 (or less) micrograms.

For most people, the pituitary gland produces sufficient HGH to retain a youthful appearance until age 35 or so. Then, somewhere between age 40-to-50, the body's ability to produce HGH declines to the point where the signs of adult growth hormone deficiency (AGHD) begin to show.

In many cases, you can reasonably look to reverse 10-to-20 years of age decline with 1 year of continual therapy by increasing your HGH.

Benefits of HGH
Abdominal Fat Reduction
Growth hormone promotes the action of insulin. When we use or increase HGH, it directs the action of insulin toward putting sugar into the cardiac muscle and nerve cells, rather then into

fat cells. By getting rid of abdominal fat, you can induce greater insulin sensitivity. Greater insulin sensitivity can help prevent, and in some cases reverse, Type 2 adult-onset diabetes.

Increase Lean Muscle

There is an average increase of 9 percent in lean muscle mass after use of HGH for 1 year, as well as reduction of 14 percent in body fat after just 6 months of HGH use.

Sex Drive

The decline of the male and female libido is directly related to the age-related declines in HGH and testosterone levels in the body. A clinical study of 302 aging adults showed that HGH and/or testosterone replacement therapy improved sexual potency and frequency in 75 percent of the men studied. Interviews with people on HGH replacement therapy indicate that almost everyone, men and women, had improvement in sexual function.

Fewer Wrinkles

Growth hormone helps with the promotion of type-2 collagen, which adds elasticity to the skin.

Healing Joints

HGH also has an anabolic effect on soft tissue such as tendons, cartilage, and other connective tissue. This signifies that old injuries can repair at an accelerated rate and with more strength due to stronger connective tissue.

Metabolic Cascade

When we age without rejuvenation, the efficiency of our overall endocrine system—thyroid, pancreas, adrenal cortal, and hypothalamic pituitary axis (HPA)—becomes tired and worn down.

In addition to this problem, a degenerative metabolic cascade takes place within the body as less hormone/messengers are produced. The receptor sites also start to lag and some become switched off; in menopause some disappear altogether. Thus, the receptor sites that serve as target areas for some hormone messengers are no longer there.

HGH has a very potent anabolic effect (protein synthesis/ tissue building), which can cause an increase in the number of cells and the enlargement of muscle cells. Restoring, retuning, and maintaining youthful hormone levels help to jumpstart tired, worn receptors. Because GH precursors rejuvenate on a cellular level through cell division, the overall effect of systemic endocrine rejuvenation has a long-lasting list of benefits.

Thus, it is essential that doctor-administered protocols, with the help of doctor's assistants for monitoring therapies are followed properly. Proper and timely dosage administration along with guidance in nutrition, adds synergy with gratifying, satisfying results.

If you decide to take HGH, the main thing is to make sure you are taking the most natural form of bio-identical HGH, so that it is all natural and of the highest quality. Consult your physician or an anti-aging specialist for the most natural bio-identical HGH available.

A better approach depending on your age and level or HGH might be to first take supplements, do exercises, and other natural methods that boost the growth hormones naturally.

Fasting is highly effective in raising HGH levels if done right. Tests conducted on lab mice have shown that regular caloric restriction actually prolongs their lifespan compared to those that had everything to eat. Fasting puts the body in a survival mode, and induces the body to release HGH to give it added strength to ride out the induced "stress" from fasting. Regular fasting for a period of 24 hours every week or 2 is a good practice because it helps the body detoxify, cleanses the bowels, and rests the body as well.

While fasting is also known to increase HGH, this is one technique that should be used sparingly. If you have a history or a risk of anorexia or bulimia, you should not fast as this can trigger the problem.

BOOSTING HGH NATURALLY

There are ways to boost your HGH levels naturally. Here are just a few.

1. **Get more sleep:** Getting eight hours of sleep is the general rule of thumb. "Not getting enough sleep regularly can lower the amount of growth hormone your body produces daily," says Walter Thompson, Ph.D., director of the Center for Sports Medicine, Science and Technology at Georgia State University in Atlanta.

   Even though excess sleep won't necessarily increase the amount of growth hormone your body secretes, constantly burning your midnight oil could be suppressing how efficiently your body distributes growth hormone during the course of the day. Keeping normal sleeping habits may let you tap into a more consistent amount of growth hormone that your bones never get a chance to utilize when sleep-deprived. Sleep is when the highest levels of fat burning and muscle recovery occur, so make it a priority.

2. **Smarter eating habits:** Focus on eating six or seven smaller meals during your day instead of three or four larger ones. Also, eating larger meals with a high glycemic index forces the body to release a higher amount of insulin into the system to help with digestion. This causes a reaction in your body to both store body fat and inhibit or slow down growth hormone being released throughout your bloodstream. One way to avoid this is to consume other low-sugar foods that will prevent and slow down the release of insulin.

   When the anterior pituitary gland is able to function at optimal levels, it speeds up the amount of growth hormone released and pumped into your system. This can be achieved by training right, eating right, sleeping right, and keeping your stress to a minimum.

3. **Pre-workout food:** Food Researchers have discovered that consuming a protein-carbohydrate meal two hours prior to working out and another meal immediately afterward elicited a significant increase in both growth hormone and testosterone within the bloodstream. Researchers at UCLA found that subjects who exercised with partially digested food in their stomachs experienced up to a 54 percent decrease in the production of growth hormone. Subjects who were fed strictly carbohydrates prior to a workout still experienced a lower production of growth hormone by up to 24 percent.

4. **Get the most from your training:** A recent study in the Journal of Applied Physiology found that the frequency and amount of growth hormone the body secretes is relative to the intensity of your workout. Subjects who exercised at a higher intensity experienced greater and more frequent releases of growth hormone after their workouts.

To get the maximum amount of growth hormone released from your training and fitness exercises, make sure that the duration and intensity of your exercise regiment is high enough to generate a response. A good standard to follow is keeping your workouts focused on short-burst, high-intensity, anaerobic stretching exercises and maintaining a pace that lasts at least 20–30 minutes. Sprinting hills, swimming, interval cycling, or cardio-boxing and other exercises that cause you to be completely out of breath will also achieve this result. Research shows that intense anaerobic exercise like weights can increase HGH levels by as much as 500%. Try also conducting intense full-body muscle exercises such as push-ups, pull-ups, and squats. These exercises encourage the body' s neuro-endocrine response which also promotes HGH release.

5. **Supplements:** It has been reported that taking the supplement acid glycine immediately before you work out can mildly stimulate the release of growth hormone, but only when taken as a supplement. But if you try to get the same effect by consuming glycine-rich foods such as poultry or milk prior to exercise, this will only inhibit growth hormone by causing you to exercise on a full stomach, plus the glycine doesn't get absorbed in the same way.

   Being introduced into the body in the presence of additional amino acids forces the glycine to compete for transport across the blood-brain barrier, diminishing its effect on the growth hormone levels. The only way glycine can cause a reaction is when taken in isolated supplement form, preferably on an empty stomach to speed up absorption and prevent outside interference from other amino acids.

6. **Don't pig out before bed:** Never eat a large meal within two hours of going to sleep. The reasoning ties into avoiding the same insulin surges you're trying to prevent during the day before a workout, but this abstention is especially important before bedtime.

   The body releases the greatest amount of growth hormone during the first two hours of sleep. Having excess insulin within the system after a large meal suppresses this higher output of growth hormone, preventing your body from taking advantages of it as you rest.

   Nighttime also seems to be the best time to take additional supplements to increase the flow of growth hormone. UCLA researchers have found that taking the amino acid arginine and orthinine together on an empty stomach right before bedtime can boost growth hormone levels significantly depending on dosage. Also the sleep aid 5-hydroxy tryptophan, a safer derivative of tryptophan, used to encourage drowsiness also helps the brain release growth hormone.

A Shortcut

As I mentioned in the weight loss chapter there is a shortcut to jump-start your anti-aging goals. Many anti-aging doctors I have spoken with (even one that is listed in Suzanne Sommers book) are starting to first put people on the HCG 500 calorie diet protocol for 21 days because they said most of the hormones like HGH, Testosterone and others that people are deficient in end up getting rebalanced and reset after a phase of HCG. The best way to know is to get the proper blood tests to see where your different hormones are at and where you are lacking. Then after going on HCG get another set of blood tests and you will notice the major difference and improvement. This is the shortest distance to the same anti-aging goals, weight loss and hormonal balance/ restoration for those that are up to it and at the same time want to remove stubborn fat deposits.

Chapter 10

Teeth

"Whether you think you can or think you cannot, either way you are right."
—Henry Ford

I first got interested in natural remedies to heal teeth when I was in Indonesia on a speaking engagement; I suddenly had the most vicious toothache. It was so bad I could not sleep night after night. I finally went online (at least I had an internet connection) and found natural remedies for toothaches and an abscessed tooth. One of the quick cures was to chew on a clove of garlic. This amazingly worked and I was fine for the rest of the trip—keeping my sanity. I realized that garlic works like a natural antibiotic killing bacteria, infections and works as good as a painkiller in most cases. I was determined now to find out more about natural ways to cure tooth problems, especially if one does not want to go through the traditional and expensive westernized forms of dental or has no access to it. It is not necessary in many cases. Ancient people and tribes had wisdom in certain areas that far surpass our modern-day science and practices in many areas.

I discovered that one of the greatest discoveries on how to cure tooth problems and cavities naturally has been overlooked—as if on purpose.

Dr. Price (a Harvard Professor) was one of the greatest pioneers in this field of tooth cures. His amazing discoveries based on ancient wisdom from indigenous cultures across the planet—Fiji to the Swiss Alps—showed how to restore dental health without surgery or chemicals. This he did by going to many different indigenous groups the world over who showed remarkable quality of teeth. There were (at least in the early 1900s) people everywhere to be found with perfect or near-perfect teeth. Instead of 50 to 95 percent tooth decay like people in modern society, certain peoples exhibited 5 to 0 percent tooth decay! What were these people doing differently and could their habits or results be emulated? This is what Dr. Price set out to find out.

Time and time again, Dr. Price documented the tragic plight of indigenous people coming into contact with industrialization. For extended periods of time, many of these groups enjoyed a life without significant tooth decay. But with the arrival of industry and commerce, and with them—modern foods—their teeth began to degenerate. Weston Price was widely respected in his time, and frequently published in many dental journals, including several articles in the *Journal of the American Dental Association*. Why have his wise words been forgotten, and what did he teach us?

The modern day way to keep teeth supposedly protected from decay and cavities is to brush and floss daily, which has not seemed to stem the increase in dental problems in this century or the last. Brushing and flossing in and of themselves are not wrong but they do not cure the problem. If brushing, flossing, massive fluoridation campaigns, and dental surgery were effective in preventing tooth decay, it would not get worse over time. It would stay the same, or get better. Most ancient people never knew about such things as brushing and flossing. One of the problems with this line of thinking is that most of the toothpaste recommended today contains fluoride.

Fluoride is the smallest negative particle and destroys enzyme molecules at very low concentrations. Fluoride actually destroys 83 of the enzymes in the body. The mechanism and process by which it destroys these enzymes has been proven by X-ray studies. Fluoride breaks up the hydrogen bonds that keep your mouth and teeth intact. It is extremely poisonous unleashing positive hydrogen bonds in enzymes and proteins. Fluoride also detaches the gum tissues forming 1-to-8 mm deep pockets. Fluoride is a nerve poison that causes cavities.

According to Dr. Judd,*(a Ph.D., Chemist and professor of Chemistry for over 33 years, and a Researcher in the industry)*, *"To avoid fluoride is to prevent more than 114 ailments … These 114 **medical side effects** extend all the way from cancers down to headaches **caused by 1 ppm fluoride in the water.** Thirteen of these side effects are proven by a double blind study on 60 patients by 12 physicians, 1 pharmacist and 1 attorney."*

Tooth decay is the #1 disease in the modern world—simply brushing, flossing, and using fluoride treatments cannot stop it. As a result, people continue to shell out cash to their dentists while their oral health deteriorates. Dental greats, Weston Price and Melvin Page have proven this. There are highly effective cavity halting and preventing protocols, along with X-ray proof of cavities healed from some of these steps in this chapter. Our bodies cannot afford denial any longer because, "It is low or no energy and unhealthy *store food* that has given us *store teeth.*"

To see your teeth go from natural to super natural health, first, stop using all toothpastes, gels, and rinses that contain fluoride and glycerin. Even the most "natural" toothpastes contain glycerin that coats the teeth preventing re-enameling. This subject is not widely talked about in the natural healing of teeth. The information here may very well save you a lot of pain and money. We will see how eating a certain way can not only save and restore your teeth but even possibly cause the re-enameling of your teeth!

There is a natural way to remineralize your teeth and even heal cavities, using proper nutrition. Many people can avoid and limit dental treatments while bringing more balance and health to their body. No longer should we accept dental surgery or the dangerous chemical fluoride as our only hope and solution for tooth decay.

Using nutrition, Dr. Weston A. Price reduced the rate of tooth decay 250 times in 17 individuals who had severe tooth decay. In this group, approximately half of all teeth had been affected by decay prior to Price's nutritional program. After the program, only two new cavities formed within a 3-year time period putting the rate of reoccurrence at 0.4 percent.[1]

THREE IMPORTANT FOOD FACTORS

Dr. Price documented that both water-soluble and fat-soluble vitamins are missing from our modern diets. Of particular note, is the near complete absence of fat-soluble vitamins in our modern diet. Without eating special foods you can be susceptible to tooth decay, gum disease, and other diseases and you do not have to always consume large amounts of them, but frequently, and enough to fill your body's needs.

---

[1] Raw grass-fed dairy including raw organic eggs, raw milk, raw cheese, raw cream, and butter. Dr. Judd says, *"Unless one furnishes extra calcium daily in their diet, that person will be sacrificing his/her teeth. Dietary calcium is absolutely necessary for good teeth and supplements alone are not sufficient."*

Eating special foods with fat-soluble vitamins won't cure tooth decay in themselves, but they are a part of the cure.

Special Foods That Help Heal Teeth

Some of you may be totally opposed to the idea of any dairy, especially if you are a vegan. I understand your reasoning as I also cut off milk and dairy until I understood the difference between pasteurized dairy, which really is harmful, and raw dairy, and how the ancients had near perfect teeth. There are two extreme lines of thought on the subject of dairy. Normally, most dairy is bad because it causes mucus and other diseases in the body when pasteurized, which is why even our kids stopped drinking it. Then I discovered that many vegans, raw foodists, and health enthusiasts in general had the worst crumbling, rotting teeth and thought that this could not be what nature or the creator intended—until I found the missing ingredient. The problem is not milk itself but all the processing it goes through. Raw and organic milk and raw cheese contain live enzymes and other raw nutrients. But, once they are pasteurized, the enzymes are destroyed diminishing the vitamin content and destroying vitamins B12 and B6. The milk proteins are altered, the beneficial bacteria killed, and the milk is no longer a natural food but more of a highly processed junk food that many rightfully claim causes allergies, heart disease, increases tooth decay, colic in infants, growth problems in children, osteoporosis, arthritis, and even cancer. Up until the 1920s when raw milk, raw cheese, and raw butter were readily available in the United States, the incidence of tooth problems was much lower.

Raw organic milk (especially goat milk) and raw organic goat cheese do the opposite effect. They provide the nutrients needed to reverse the decay process in teeth and help to re-mineralize the enamel.

Percentages of Teeth Attacked By Dental Caries in Primitive and Modern Groups		
Group	Primitive	Modern
Swiss	4.60	29.8
Gaelics	1.20	30.0
Eskimos	0.09	13.0
Northern Indians	0.16	21.5
Seminole Indians	4.00	40.0
Melanesians	0.38	29.0
Polynesians	0.32	21.9

ISOLATED SWISS

In 1932 when Dr. Price visited the people of the-then more remote and primitive Lötschental Valley in Switzerland, he found that no deaths had ever occurred from tuberculosis. The locals had neither physician nor dentist and no policeman or jail because they had no need for them. They didn't have a varied diet at all; only a few percent had dental problems. The demands they placed on their foods, however, were high. They only ate butter and cheese from milk from cows that had grazed freely on spring and summer grasses.

These isolated people had some of the finest physiques in all of Europe.

They had a normal design of face and dental arches when adequate nutrition was provided for both the parents and the children. They had well-developed nostrils and lacked tooth decay.

Doctor Price wrote, "The isolated Swiss children were remarkably healthy. The sturdiness of the child's life permits children to play and frolic bareheaded and barefooted even in water running down from the glacier in the late evening's chilly breezes, in weather that made us wear our overcoats and gloves and button our collars. They ate whole rye bread, summer cheese (about

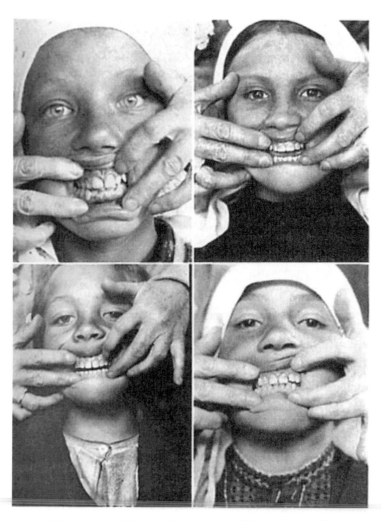

Source: "Nutrition and Physical Degeneration", By Dr. Price, Ch 3, www.
journeytoforever.org/farm_library/price/price3.html.

as large as the slice of bread), which are eaten with fresh milk of
goats or cows. Meat is eaten once a week." A delightful photo of
the children barefoot on the side of the mountain can be found on
the cover of The Price–Pottenger Nutrition Foundation's *Health
and Healing Wisdom* Journal, Winter 2006.

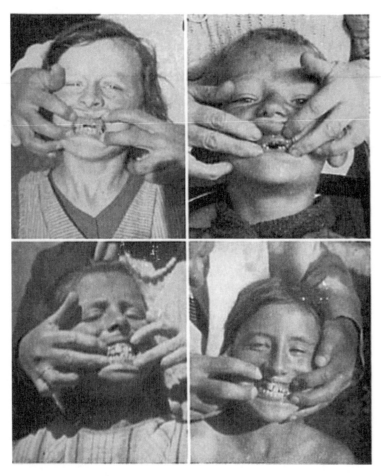

Source: "Nutrition and Physical Degeneration", By Dr. Price, Ch 3, www.journeytoforever.org/farm_library/price/price3.html.

Notice the difference and the degeneration with the modern diet in the teeth, facial structure and dental arches in the photos below compared to the first set of photos above.

In the modernized districts of Switzerland tooth decay is rampant. The girl in the second set of photos, upper left, is older and the one to the right is younger. They use white bread and sweets liberally. The two children below have very badly formed dental arches with crowding of the teeth. This deformity is not due to heredity.

If you are a vegan, you can still opt out of eating meat but increasing your raw dairy intake will make a huge difference!

Other special foods include:

1. Organs of sea animals: also uncooked or slightly cooked wild fish (sashimi, salmon, tuna rare or seared etc.)

2. Organs of land animals, including liver, bone marrow, kidneys, pancreas, adrenal glands, and gonads. Also organic pasture-raised lamb, chicken rare or medium rare (this of course is for non-vegans).

Making bone-broths like a fish stew broth is very mineralizing for teeth. Bones and other parts of the body of animals can and should also be utilized. A lion or dog will chew and suck on a bone for hours. Because it's bored? No. Because of the necessary nutrients to be found inside like when we give bones to our dogs (who usually has much better teeth than we do. Without brushing!) Bones, fish-heads, and all kinds of animal parts can be used for making stock that we then use as a base for a soup or other dishes for flavor. Fish parts need only boil for about an hour, other types of stock may simmer for a whole day. Dr. Price found that one characteristic of groups containing a high immunity to tooth decay is that they ate regularly from two of these three food categories.

Our modern diet is so lacking in these special foods—they are not consumed in regular amounts—so it is no wonder why our bodies degenerate. Until we change the way we live, and return to more natural and life-building foods, the trend of tooth decay worsening with age, will continue.

FREEDOM FROM TOOTH DECAY

This is just a starter chapter on your journey to learn how you can be free of tooth decay, and avoid unpleasant root canals. Our teeth can rebuild themselves, and cover themselves over with a hard and glassy layer, if we give ourselves the right kind of nutrition. You can minimize your tooth decay, yes even prevent it entirely and even heal it once a cavity has formed, if you make the right choices for yourself based on the knowledge of decay-free indigenous peoples.

RE-GROWING YOUR TEETH

Your body is made to reproduce. You have a new skeleton every 3 months. Every 4 weeks you re-grow new skin. Given the right conditions and nutrients, your teeth enamel can re-grow, teeth can heal, and cavities can disappear. The Inuits, for example, in the Arctic often have severely worn teeth temporarily from chewing on leather and from small bits of sand and grit that collect when they eat fish dried in the wind. But due to their excellent diet, their teeth constantly repair themselves to such a point that the tooth pulp chambers and nerves are very well protected. This is not evident with Inuits who leave behind their ancient natural diet and switch to a modern food diet.

Also, I have noticed that adequate amounts of vitamin C also help the teeth. At least 1,000 mg of vitamin C daily along with vitamin D really help to strengthen the teeth against decay. Another incredible product I have discovered is Biosil containing silica.

SILICA

Calcium, of course, is important for your bone growth and formation but even more important is the mineral called silica (silicon dioxide). You don't have enough of this mineral in your diet and you can take a ton of calcium and brush your teeth five times a day and still lose your teeth, just like your hair in the shower, as you get older without it.

The formula called Biosil is known to provide a sufficient nutritional support for your tooth repair/growth. It will improve your teeth, bones, and connective tissue, and will also help calcium metabolize in your body (without it most of your calcium will go right through you, especially if you take it as a part of a common multivitamin formula). *According to the makers of BioSil (Si[OH]$_4$) it is 20,000 times more soluble than silica (SiO$_2$—found in horsetail and colloidal gels) and 2.5 times more bioavailable than other forms of silicon according to the makers of Biosil.*

STIMULATING TEETH TO RE-GROW

A team of Alberta researchers applied for a patent that claims they created a miniature device to stimulate the jaw bones and gums around an affected tooth. Using low-intensity ultrasound technology, **they claim they have been able to regrow the root of a tooth and stimulate tooth growth and repair.** The wireless design of the ultrasound transducer means the miniscule device will be able to fit comfortably inside a patient's mouth while packed with biocompatible materials. The unit will be easily mounted on an orthodontic or "braces" bracket or even a plastic removable crown. The team also designed an energy sensor that will ensure the power is reaching the target area of the teeth roots within the bone. TEC Edmonton is the University of Alberta's exclusive tech transfer service provider. They filed the first patent recently in the United States. Currently, the research team is finishing the system-on-a-chip and hopes to complete the miniaturized device soon. The process invigorates the inside of our teeth for increased healthier tissue.

Dr. El-Bialy is an orthodontist and one of the inventors of the ultrasound stimulation device with credentials from the University of Alabama and Tanta University. He says, "**The added growth of dentin bolsters the enamel as it was when you were a**

younger person. In addition an increase of density in mandible bone and upper tooth support solidifies tooth roots. He goes on to say, "Our experience shows a solid bite equal to that in our teenage years. The ringing of teeth when biting down hard, which we had forgotten entirely, was back again."

Using low-intensity pulsed ultrasound (LIPUS), Dr. Tarak El-Bialy from the Faculty of Medicine and Dentistry and Drs. Jie Chen and Ying Tsui from the Faculty of Engineering have created a miniaturized system-on-a-chip that offers a non-invasive and novel way to stimulate jaw growth and dental tissue healing.

Professor Paul Sharpe, Head of the Department of Craniofacial Development, King's College London stated: "A key medical advantage of this new technology is that a living tooth can preserve the health of the surrounding tissues much better than artificial prosthesis. Teeth are living, and they are able to respond to a person's bite. They move, and in doing so they maintain the health of the surrounding gums and teeth."

"If the root is broken, it can now be fixed," said El-Bialy. "And because we can regrow the teeth root, a patient could have his own tooth rather than foreign objects in his mouth."

Although the technology may not be available for many, the basic idea is using a low frequency ultrasound source. Because you can't buy a real ultrasound machine unless you are a physician, here are some possible alternatives.

Another option is a Novasonic massager that can generate a sound vibration of 20,000 Hertz. It is not your regular massager and all you have to do is slightly touch the skin and you can feel the sound waves go deep within your body. So basically what you would do is apply the sound waves from the device to the teeth and gums for a few minutes every day and get a gentle but thorough massage this way to stimulate growth. If you try another type of ultrasound massager make sure you get one that only generates only 1-to-2 mHz as others can generate up to 3-to-5 mHz frequency but they reportedly are not as effective going only ⅛ -inch to ¼ -inch deep as opposed to the preferred lower but more effective frequency of 1-to-2 mHz.

Other teeth cleaning options that I researched for optimum cleaning instead of regular tooth paste would be toothsoap (www. toothsoap.com). Otherwise you can always make your own with all or some of these ingredients:

1. Unprocessed raw coconut oil (also swishing this for a minute a day will help clean and pull out junk from the teeth)
2. Tea tree oil
3. Baking soda ⅟₁₀ part
4. Extra virgin olive Oil (2 part)
5. Spearmint or peppermint oil (⅟₁₀ part)
6. Unprocessed sea salt or Himalayan salt (⅟₅₀ part)
7. Eucalyptus oil (⅟₁₀ part)
8. Food-grade hydrogen peroxide (⅟₁₀ part)

I hope I have awakened your curiosity and that you will start to adjust your diet to start re-pairing your teeth as you also delve much deeper into this subject realizing that like every other part of your body, your teeth were not meant to decay the way they do today in our modern world. For more information on this subject and supplements for curing tooth decay, the truth about root canals and what to use for brushing, and other natural tooth remedies, I recommend a great book called, *Cure Tooth Decay Today* by Ramiel Nagel along with the writings of Dr. Price entitled *Nutrition and Physical Degeneration*.

Chapter 11

The Highest Power Source

"Surely God would not have created such a being as man,
with an ability to grasp the infinite, to exist only for a day!
No, no, man was made for immortality."
—Abraham Lincoln

Though modern man has achieved many historic breakthroughs making life much easier in many ways, we have also lost a great deal of ancient wisdom. In Okinawa, Japan there are people who live very long, having some of the longest life spans on earth. In fact some of the longest life spans are in this area of the world where it is common for people to be walking around at 120 years old exercising, working, and enjoying life—living up to 120 years of age. Some attribute this to their diet high in coral calcium from the ocean, exercise and peace of mind as they live more connected to how we were supposed to live as far as health and rest go, limiting the stresses and toxic lifestyle of some of the larger cities.

A group called the Essenes who lived in the desert in Israel moved away from the city and lived and ate extremely healthy. They also regularly did cleansing techniques like colonics for both physical and spiritual cleansing. They were some of the healthiest people of their day.

Even the Native Americans of North America, if you look at the early pictures looked very slim, muscular, confident and healthy, until they began to eat westernized food and embraced a more indoor sedentary lifestyle. This has resulted in many sicknesses and social problems that they never knew before. They were also much more connected to nature and the land in the old days as much of this ancient wisdom and health and joy of living have been lost in modern times. Today the average Native American looks physically different from their ancestors who lived off of the land. There are some that are starting on the journey to rediscover the beauty and healing life of eating and living more in a way that is connected with how they were meant to live.

There is an ancient and well-documented story about a Hebrew man named, Daniel, who worked for a foreign king. He was offered the best meats—fit for a king. He asked instead if he and his friends could eat a different diet even for a few weeks—not eating the king's meat but raw, healthy vegetables—foods that shocked the king and the royal court. After the few weeks, these Hebrews were smarter, stronger, more vibrant than that of the others in the king's palace. Whether or not they were always pure vegetarians is not mentioned as this diet was for a few weeks to prove the different effects healthier food have on the body and mind, but it does shows that even in ancient times people have known the power and benefits of eating high-energy super foods.

Daniel, who held a high government position also became a spiritual leader defying the powers of the day as he demonstrated a higher power source than others in that nation as he prayed only to the Creator and not the manmade images of the day which almost cost him his life. Daniel also went on a 21-day fast of only vegetables and was visited by an angel at the end of the fast. It is possible to eat in a certain way for a specific period of time or even abstain from food for a season and go from a natural to a supernatural state in a very short time. When you are in this supernatural state you tend to be much more aware of the spiritual world; your sense of discernment or intuition is heightened. You start to have a keen sense about things that prove to be true, and most of all you seem to access the supernatural world much easier. People groups all over the world have used fasting to access the spiritual world. But when you also simply eat and live in a certain way as part of a daily lifestyle, you can enjoy the benefits of natural to supernatural health, as Daniel did.

Another ancient prophet named Ezekiel was given a divine recipe from the Creator and told to live off of this special bread for years which he did. Today this same bread is available in health food stores across the nation; it is known as Ezekiel bread. It has no flour, but contains barley, lentils, oats, and wheat. It is understandable why it sustained him; the bread contains vital nutrients and superfoods. Many spiritual giants had certain lifestyle differences in their food choices, connection to the outdoors and nature, quiet times to connect to the Creator and other patterns that we see again as they seem driven to a non-toxic life in the natural leading to a supernatural life or a spiritual life that leads them to a healthier natural life.

WHAT IS THE HIGHEST POWER SOURCE?

There are many power sources but like everything—high levels of power and low levels of power exist. The highest power source would be whatever created power to begin with. Creation is extremely powerful. Eating freshly created raw food has a power source. Hanging out in the mountains or on the ocean gives power. People meditate or pray to different things claiming a certain level of power. The Creator who made the creation is the Highest Power Source. The source of all things is the greatest power.

Throughout history some of the most ancient people groups on the earth have known this truth. The Chinese and the first

22 emperors would worship the Creator—the Creator of Heaven and Earth. They would offer sacrifices to the creator whose name in Chinese is Sheng Ti. In Korean they worshipped the Creator whose name in Korean is Haniim. The Hawaiians, the Hebrews, Native Americans and people around the world worshipped the Creator that made everything seen and unseen. Another common practice was that they would offer a sacrifice of an animal known as a blood sacrifice. This seems very strange and even repulsive to most people in the modern world. Why would blood be so key in accessing the Creator? Well we know that life is in the blood. If you lose your blood you will die. The ancient peoples across continents and tribes worldwide always believed that the Creator required and would be pleased by sacrificial blood.

I discovered in researching this that the same story of Creation basically spread to the entire world—mankind started off pretty much perfect and even superhuman compared to today. Mankind lost its superhuman and naturally supernatural state when it sinned against the Creator. Instead of loving and worshipping the Creator, mankind started to believe more in the serpent and Creation, and that it did not need to love and thank the Creator; mankind assumed he was just as good without the Creator's help—turning away from the ways of the Creator. Once this occurred, the process of death, murder, theft, sickness, toxic living and every negative thing known to man occurred. Ever since, humankind has been attempting to return to the Creator. Blood sacrifice was what the Creator asked the first humans to do to reconnect with the Highest Power Source according to the most ancient texts around the world as even recorded in the ancient book of Genesis. An innocent animal would have to suffer and die for a guilty person to be connected back to the Creator as blood is symbolic for life on account of man's sin against the Creator.

What is amazing was that the idea of animal sacrifice started to change over the past 20 centuries and now is not as common in many cultures, which I am sure the animals are thankful for—not only because it seems to our natural minds like a sad and cruel thing to kill an innocent animal but someone changed this dilemma in the human condition. The greatest spiritual being to ever walk the earth changed this entire process. The Magi, people who could read and study the stars (the wisemen of the east), began to pick up that something big was going to happen when the ultimate supernatural being came on the scene whose original ancient name is Yeshua. These were star gazers from ethnic tribes to the eastern part of the Middle East. They followed the exact location of where the star would lead them to pay homage to this One that would change it all—to reconnect man back to the Creator. They always knew that a messiah figure would come and change the process reversing the negative consequences of the human condition, but now they were able to map out exactly when and where the Messiah would appear due to their knowledge of the stars. Their search landed them in the nation of Israel that was then under Roman occupation. They told the king at the time why they were there—to find the Messiah that was about to be born. This must have been a pretty big deal. They found Yeshua whose life later split time in half as we know it from B.C. to A.D. All this He did, the only 100% pure, non-toxic Sinless One with one act of self-sacrifice becoming the connection for man to reconnect to the Creator. This one act of allowing Himself to be the final sacrifice that would abolish the need for animal sacrifice practiced by so many cultures waiting for the Messiah would take man's guilt away and restore peace and harmony in his spirit, soul, mind, and body once and for all for whoever was willing to believe it and tap into this new supernatural life accessing the Highest Power Source.

It is recorded that when Yeshua died that He took on all of humanity's original rebellion, pride and sin against the Creator. Again the spiritual law of the cosmos was that only a 100%

innocent sinless blood as a sacrifice could once and for all reverse mankind's toxic, self-destructive pattern. It is also recorded in the annals of history that at Yeshua's death there was a major earthquake and some type of solar eclipse and that this Messiah even resurrected from the dead against all odds. The authorities of the time could not handle the fact that the Highest Power source was in their midst as they saw Yeshua as a threat since no one else possessed such supernatural miraculous abilities and exuded such energy, power and love. Yeshua was known to heal, forgive, and even resurrect people who had died. When He resurrected Himself it proved that there was no other higher power source that one could experience.

This act of love completely removed the wall between humans and the Highest Power Source, the Creator Himself. No longer was an animal blood sacrifice needed for the tribes of the earth to access the Creator, the Messiah became this sacrifice once and for all. Now humans could once again be purified in soul, mind, body and spirit from mankind's toxic and self-destructive nature both spiritually and physically and reconnect with the Creator.

All you have to do now to access the Highest Power Source and experience this incredible high level sheer peace in mind, body, soul, and spirit is to tell the Creator that you thank Him for sending Yeshua as a sacrifice so that you could have a direct relationship with the Creator. Believe that it really happened and acknowledge that the Creator is the source of all life and through Yeshua you choose to invite Him into your entire being turning away from low level living and all inferior power sources that distract and cut you off from the ultimate true source of love, joy, peace and health, the Creator of Heaven and Earth. Invite Him in today!

As you begin your journey from natural to supernatural health, may you also find a connection with the Creator today and experience health not just in your body and mind, but in your soul, bringing you a new joy and life.

As you start to change your eating habits and lifestyle while cleansing your body of harmful toxins and reduce stress while losing excess weight, you body will start to be transformed into a beautiful sculpture of youthful vibrant energy as your new life will start to unravel opening up dormant creativity propelling you with a newfound joy to fully discover and achieve your destiny!

I am cheering you on as you go from "Natural to Super Natural Health!"

Resource Guide to Super Natural Health

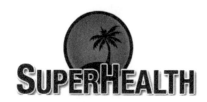

SuperHealth
2675 W. S.R. 89A, #464
Sedona, AZ 86336
Toll Free: 1-800-266-5564
Website: superhealthvitamins.com
Committed to achieving Super Health!

SuperHealth vitamins and supplements are of the highest quality including organic, kosher and whole-food products for those seeking super health in every way. Many of the products found in the book, *Natural to Super Natural Health* are manufactured for and distributed by *SuperHealth*.

Some of the unique supplements *SuperHealth* offers are:
Organic Spirulina, Organic Grass Juice, Organic Green Veggie, Organic Blue Green Algae, Organic Fruit and Greens, Organic Psyllium, Organic Berry Powder, Organic Garlic, 100% Organic Fiber, Chlorella, Super-Food Based Multi-Vitamins, Echinacea/Goldenseal, CoQ10, Immunity Formula, Brain Formula, 100%, Panax Ginseg, Hair, Skin and Nails, Reversatrol, Saw Palmetto, MSM, Double Strength Probiotics, and so much more. *SuperHealth* also offers premium supplement categories such as antioxidants, enzymes, amino acids, B vitamins, herbs, joint health, essential fatty acids, minerals, and specialty blend formulas.

SuperHealth is committed to and believes in offering only the highest quality, nutrient-rich whole-food ingredients, the reason that whenever possible many of the raw materials are certified organic, kosher, food based and pesticide/herbicide free.

About the Author

David Herzog is a nutrition coach, a powerful peak performance motivational speaker and life coach. David also works in conjunction with the premier supplement company, *SuperHealth* that is manufactured for and distributed by *www.superhealthvitamins. com*. He is also the founder of *David Herzog Entertainment LLC.* David has given 1000's of lectures and television/radio interviews during his speaking tours. He has also helped actors and entertainers, presidents and vice presidents of nations and other heads of state worldwide, leading businessmen, health and sports professionals, has been invited to the White House and has shared his keys and insights at the U.N. His work as a motivational speaker (mixed with lots of comedy), has taken him across North and South America, the Caribbean, Europe, Asia, Australia, New Zealand, South Pacific Islands, Africa, Middle East, India, Sri Lanka and even among the native tribes of the world helping people from every sphere of society achieve their highest potential.

Apart from his very exciting schedule he is also involved in acting, comedy, and writing movie scripts and TV shows. Currently David also is also working on several new cutting edge books.

Other than his passion for super health, David's hobbies are hiking, surfing, reading, writing, singing, comedy, nature exploration, investing and travelling the entire globe to the far away places and tribes many westerners have never visited. His favorite hobby is spending time with his family and loved ones. He is based in his hometown of Sedona Arizona, one of the healthiest and most spiritual towns in America.

To contact David or book him on a television or radio show, for an interview or for a seminar please contact:

David Herzog Entertainment LLC
2675 W. 89A, #464
Sedona, AZ 86336
superhealthdh@aol.com

Websites:
davidherzogbook.com
superhealthvitamins.com
davidherzog.net
davidherzog.com

Additional Copies of *Natural to Super Natural Health*
Additional copies of *Natural to Super Natural Health* may be ordered directly from davidherzogbook.com. You can also call toll free at 1-800-BOOK-LOG.

Glossary of Terms

Acetylcholine: A chemical produced by the body vital for healthy brain function. Acetylcholine improves memory, concentration, and cognition, by increasing blood flow to the brain.

Amino Acids: The building blocks that make up proteins. Humans need 20 different amino acids to function properly. Some are made by the body. Others, called essential amino acids, must be obtained from foods.

Antioxidant: Substances, like vitamins A, C, E, and beta-carotene, that protect your body from the damage of oxidation caused by free radicals.

Chlorella: Chlorella is a powerful detoxification aid for heavy metals and other pesticides. Numerous research projects in the U.S. and Europe indicate that chlorella can also aid the body in breaking down persistent hydrocarbon and metallic toxins such as mercury, cadmium and lead, DDT and PCB while strengthening the immune system response.

Colon Therapy/Colon Hydrotherapy/Colonics: Colon therapy uses a series of filtered and temperature regulated water flushes into the colon. These water flushes cleanse and detoxify the lower intestine and aid in the reconstitution of intestinal flora. The purpose of colonics is to balance the body chemistry, eliminate toxic wastes that have accumulated, and restore proper tissue and organ function.

Detox: Body cleansing or detoxification is a alternative medicine approach which rids the body of "toxins", usually in the form of dieting, fasting, consuming exclusively, or avoiding specific foods such as fats, carbohydrates, fruits, vegetables, juices, herbs or water.

Dopamine: Dopamine is a chemical naturally produced in the body. It controls the voltage and power of your brain and its ability to process information.

EMF or Electric and Magnetic Fields: An invisible field of electro-magnetism radiated from sources such as appliances, transmission towers, cell phones and other electronic devices.

Free Radicals: An atom or molecule with at least one unpaired electron, making it unstable and reactive. When free radicals react with certain chemicals in the body, they may interfere with the ability of cells to function normally. Antioxidants can stabilize free radicals.

GABA (gamma-aminobutyric acid): GABA is a non-protein amino acid that functions as a neurotransmitter. It is the primary inhibitory neurotransmitter in the brain, and serves to cause relaxation, reduce stress, and increase alertness.

HCG (Human Chorionic Gonadotropin): A naturally occurring hormone found in the urine of pregnant women. HCG is said "to perform a metabolic recovery, where the hypothyroid is said to be reset, boosting the metabolism, and increasing the person's ability to burn fat at a much higher rate."

HGH (human growth hormone): HGH is an endocrine hormone produced by the anterior portion of the pituitary gland.

Homeopathy: Homeopathy is a medical system that uses minute doses of natural substances-called remedies-to stimulate a person's immune and defense system.

Massage: Massage is the manipulation of the superficial tissues of the human body in order to promote deep relaxation, and release tension. Recent research has proven that massage is therapeutic, and can soothe injured muscles, stimulate blood and lymphatic circulation, improve structure and function of the body, increase toxic elimination, and more.

Micronutrients: The name given to vitamins and minerals because your body needs them in small amounts. Micronutrients are vital to your body's ability to process the "macronutrients:" fats, proteins, and carbohydrates. Examples are chromium, zinc, and selenium.

Minerals: Nutrients found in the earth or water and absorbed by plants and animals for proper nutrition. Minerals are the main component of teeth and bones, and help build cells and support nerve impulses, among other things. One example is calcium.

Natural Medicine: Natural medicine or healing is the use of non-invasive and non-pharmaceutical techniques for providing wellness.

Nutrient: A nutrient is any chemical element, chemical compound, or combination of chemical elements and/or chemical compounds that contributes to bodily development or is necessary for life.

Probiotics: Probiotics are live microorganisms thought to be healthy for the host organism. Probiotics are commonly consumed as part of fermented foods with specially added active live cultures; such as in yogurt, soy yogurt, or as dietary supplements.

Serotonin: A chemical produced naturally by the body which aids in feelings of well-being, restfulness, and relaxation.

Spirulina: Spirulina is a microscopic blue-green algae in the shape of a perfect spiral coil, living both in sea and fresh water. It is the one of nature's richest source of vitamins, iron, protein, carbohydrates, micronutrients and beta carotene.

Supplements: Vitamins, minerals, herbs, or other substances taken orally and meant to correct deficiencies in the diet.

References

Good Teeth, Birth to Death, Gerard F. Judd, 1996, http://gerardjudd.com/affidavit.htm.

"HCG and The Weight Loss Cure," Christmas Jones, International Association for Physicians in Aesthetic Medicine, 2007, www.IAPAM.com.

"Lymphatic Immune Support," *Well Being Journal,* May/June 2000, www.wellbeingjournal.com.

Managing Nano-Bio-Info-Cogno Innovations: Converging Technologies in Society, page 144, William Sims Bainbridge, Mihail C. Roco, 2009.

"Quoting from the Schuphan Study," page 223, *The Sunfood Diet Success System,* David Wolfe, 2000.

Raw Foods Bible, page 74, Craig B. Sommers, 2007.

"Ultrasound May Help Regrow Teeth," *ScienceDaily,* June 28, 2006, www.sciencedaily.com/releases/2006/06/060628234304.htm.

ADDITIONAL RECOMMENDED READING

Cure Tooth Decay Today, Ramiel Nagel, 2008.

Jumping for Health, Morton Walker, 2005.

Nutrition and Physical Degeneration, Weston A. Price, 2008.

Rebounding to Better Health, Linda Brooks, 1997.

Younger You, Eric Braverman, 2008.

Index